HOW THINGS WORK
THE BRAIN

Other publications:

AMERICAN COUNTRY
VOYAGE THROUGH THE UNIVERSE
THE THIRD REICH
THE TIME-LIFE GARDENER'S GUIDE
MYSTERIES OF THE UNKNOWN
TIME FRAME
FIX IT YOURSELF
FITNESS, HEALTH & NUTRITION
SUCCESSFUL PARENTING
HEALTHY HOME COOKING
UNDERSTANDING COMPUTERS
LIBRARY OF NATIONS
THE ENCHANTED WORLD
THE KODAK LIBRARY OF CREATIVE PHOTOGRAPHY
GREAT MEALS IN MINUTES
THE CIVIL WAR
PLANET EARTH
COLLECTOR'S LIBRARY OF THE CIVIL WAR
THE EPIC OF FLIGHT
THE GOOD COOK
WORLD WAR II
HOME REPAIR AND IMPROVEMENT
THE OLD WEST

COVER
Angiography, the process that traces blood flow, shows how greedy the normal adult brain is. It receives one-fifth of the body's total supply, yet accounts for only one-fiftieth of the body's weight.

HOW THINGS WORK

THE BRAIN

TIME-LIFE BOOKS

ALEXANDRIA, VIRGINIA

Library of Congress Cataloging-in-Publication Data

The brain
     p. cm. – (How things work)
  Includes index.
  ISBN 0-8094-7854-4 (trade)
  ISBN 0-8094-7855-2 (lib.)
  1. Brain—Popular works.
  I. Time-Life Books. II. Series.
  QP376.B6933   1990
  152—dc20   90-42780
                                   CIP

How Things Work was produced by
ST. REMY PRESS

PRESIDENT	Pierre Léveillé
PUBLISHER	Kenneth Winchester

Staff for THE BRAIN

Editor	Carolyn Jackson
Senior Art Director	Diane Denoncourt
Art Director	Odette Sévigny
Assistant Editor	Daniel McBain
Contributing Editor	George Daniels
Research Editor	Fiona Gilsenan
Researcher	Hayes Jackson
Picture Editor	Chris Jackson
Designer	Chantal Bilodeau
Illustrators	Maryse Doray, Nicolas Moumouris, Robert Paquet, Maryo Proulx
Index	Christine M. Jacobs
Administrator	Natalie Watanabe
Production Manager	Michelle Turbide
Coordinator	Dominique Gagné
Systems Coordinator	Jean-Luc Roy

Time-Life Books Inc. is a wholly owned subsidiary of
THE TIME INC. BOOK COMPANY

President and Chief Executive Officer	Kelso F. Sutton
President, Time Inc. Books Direct	Christopher T. Linen

TIME-LIFE BOOKS INC.

EDITOR	George Constable
Director of Design	Louis Klein
Director of Editorial Resources	Phyllis K. Wise
Director of Photography and Research	John Conrad Weiser
PRESIDENT	John M. Fahey Jr.
Senior Vice Presidents	Robert M. DeSena, Paul R. Stewart, Curtis G. Viebranz, Joseph J. Ward
Vice Presidents	Stephen L. Bair, Bonita L. Boezeman, Mary P. Donohoe, Stephen L. Goldstein, Juanita T. James, Andrew P. Kaplan, Trevor Lunn, Susan J. Maruyama, Robert H. Smith
New Product Development	Trevor Lunn, Donia Ann Steele
Supervisor of Quality Control	James King
PUBLISHER	Joseph J. Ward

Editorial Operations

Production	Celia Beattie
Library	Louise D. Forstall
Correspondents	Elisabeth Kraemer-Singh (Bonn); Christina Lieberman (New York); Maria Vincenza Aloisi (Paris); Ann Natanson (Rome).

THE WRITERS

Sarah Brash's work has appeared in numerous Time-Life Books series, including the *Life Science Library*, *Voyage Through the Universe*, *Planet Earth* and *Understanding Computers*.

Gina Maranto is an award-winning science journalist who has written for *Discover*, *Redbook*, *The New York Times*, and numerous other publications.

Wendy Murphy has written frequently for Time-Life Books on medical subjects. She will soon release a book on gardening.

Bryce Walker is a former writer and editor of Time-Life Books. He now works as a writer, specializing in science, travel and history topics.

THE CONSULTANTS

Rafael Cabeza is a cholinegic neurochemist at McGill University, Montreal, Québec, interested in the cellular regulation of REM sleep and REM rebound.

Mark S. Freedman is a neuroimmunologist at the Montreal Neurological Institute and is an Assistant Professor at McGill University in the Department of Neurology and Neurosurgery. His main interest is in multiple sclerosis.

Michael S. Gazzaniga is a professor of neuroscience and psychiatry at Dartmouth Medical School, NH. He is known for his studies on split-brain patients and is the author of the bestseller *Mind Matters*.

John B. Mitchell, a researcher at the Douglas Hospital Research Center, McGill University, studies the interactions between hormones, neurotransmitters and experience in the control of behavior.

Howard Mount is a neuropharmacologist at McGill University researching the interaction between excitatory amino acids and dopamine transmission.

Urs Ribary directs the Center for Neuromagnetism at the NYU Medical Center in New York City, under the supervision of department chairman Dr. R. Llinas.

For information about any Time-Life book,
please write:
Reader Information
Time-Life Customer Service
P.O. Box C-32068
Richmond, Virginia
23261-2068

© 1990 Time-Life Books Inc. All rights reserved. No part of this book may be reproduced in any form or by any electronic or mechanical means, including information storage and retrieval devices or systems, without prior written permission from the publisher, except that brief passages may be quoted for reviews. First printing. Printed in U.S.A.
Published simultaneously in Canada.
School and library distribution by Silver Burdett Company, Morristown, New Jersey.

TIME-LIFE is a trademark of Time Warner Inc. U.S.A.

CONTENTS

8 BUILDING A BRAIN

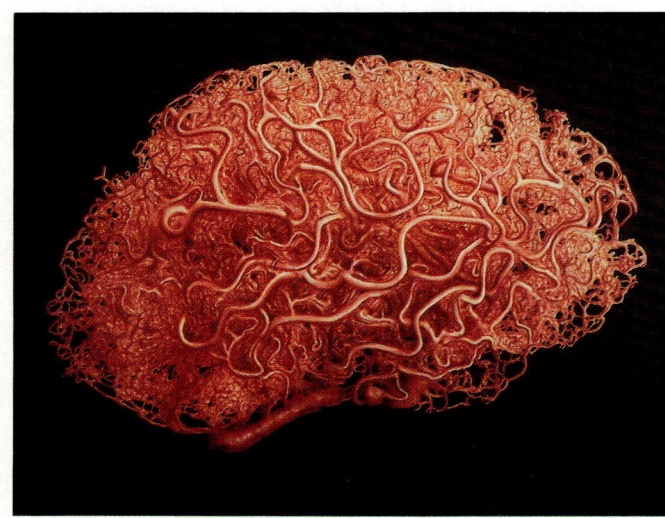
Artist's impression of the brain's blood vessel network

14 STAYING ALIVE

- 18 Running the Machine
- **24 Running on Empty**
- 27 Common Senses
- 35 Grace in Space
- **38 Motor Misfires**
- 40 Survival of the Species
- **44 The Detectives**

50 STATES OF MIND

- 52 Scattered Signals
- 56 Sleepyhead
- **58 Mind over Matter**
- **64 Time Flies**
- 67 The Stuff of Dreams
- **68 Too Little. . . Too Much**
- 74 ¿Siesta? ¡Sí!

76 MOOD, MOLECULES AND MADNESS

- 79 Feelings
- **84 Love's Elixir**
- **88 Face Value**
- 91 Stressed Out
- **96 Put on a Happy Face**
- 98 Hooking the Brain
- **104 Natural Highs**

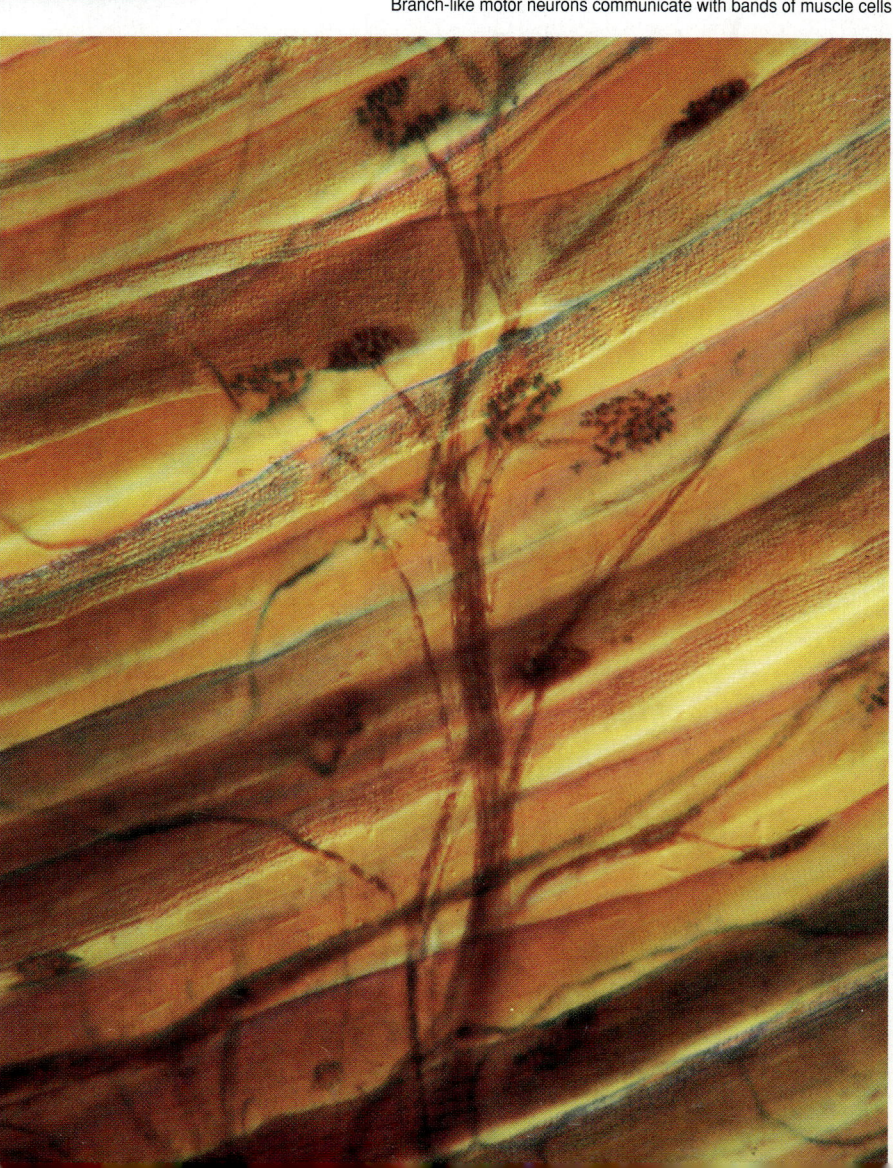
Branch-like motor neurons communicate with bands of muscle cells

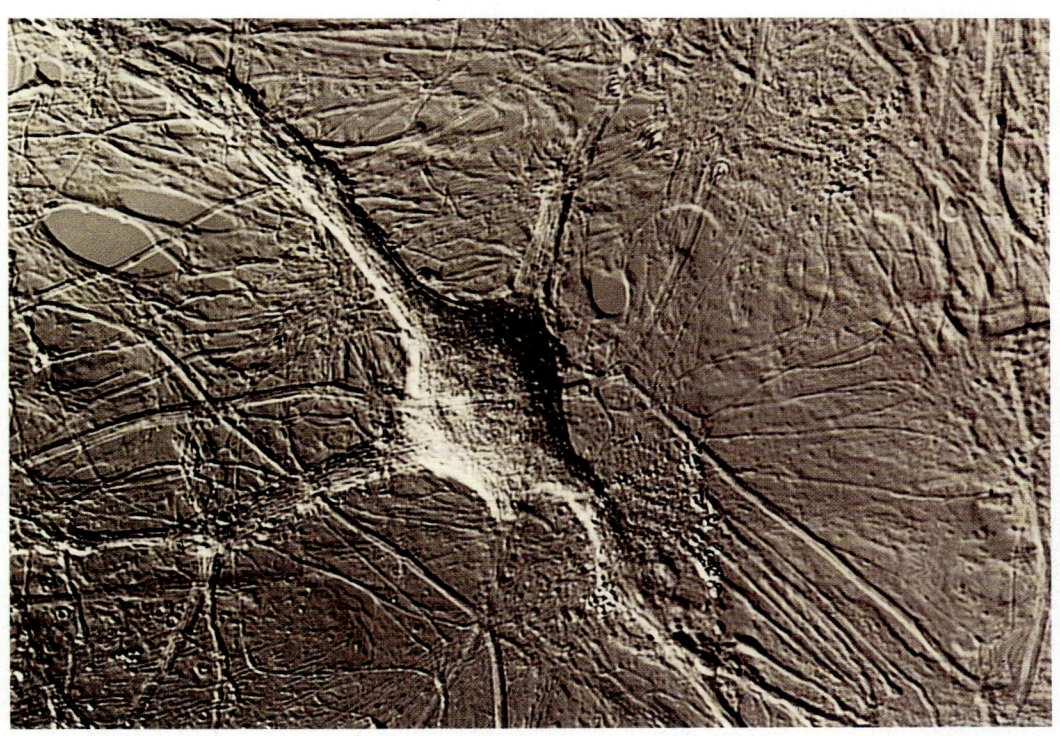

A healthy adult brain cell

106 NETWORKS OF BRILLIANCE

- 108 Neural Nets
- 110 **Rajan the Pi-Man**
- 115 Beyond the Here and Now
- 116 **The Agony of Alzheimer's**
- 122 **Of Two Minds**
- 124 Leaping Logic
- 127 Grade A Brain
- 128 **Free Thinking**

134 GIANT STEPS

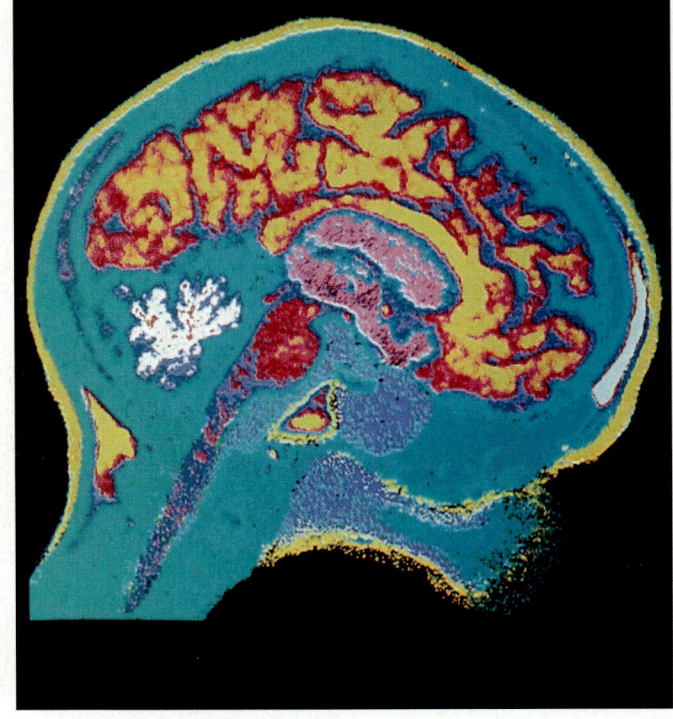

Color tissue scan of an Alzheimer's patient

- 140 INDEX
- 143 PICTURE AND ILLUSTRATION CREDITS
- 144 ACKNOWLEDGMENTS

During its third month of development, the translucent fetus begins to take on recognizable features. The still-sightless eyes are migrating into place from the sides of the head. Brain cells—or neurons—at times grow at the astounding rate of 250,000 per minute. Even at this early stage, slow waves of brain activity can be detected.

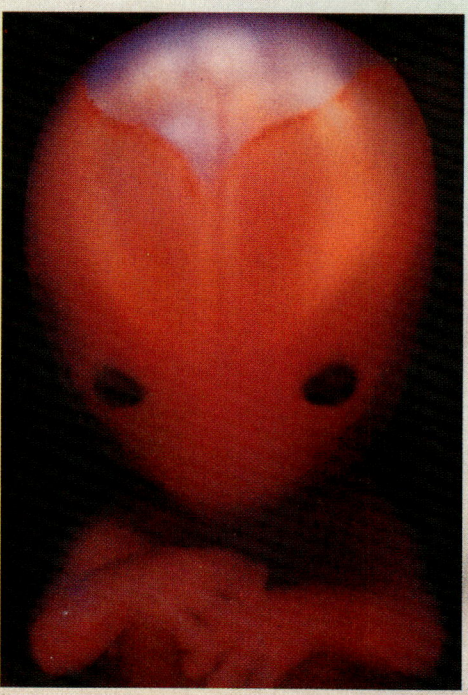

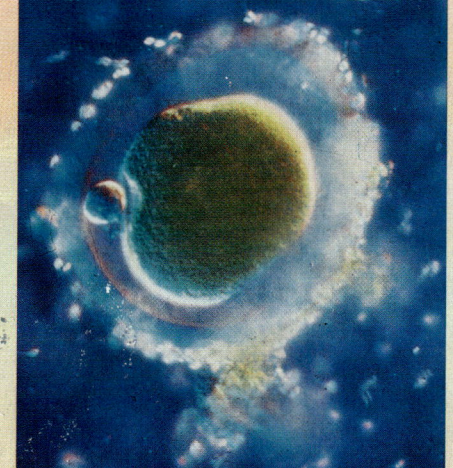

At this moment, when the human ovum is fertilized by a sperm, cell division—and life—has begun. Two hollow balls of cells develop very quickly and the area where they touch thickens. Eighteen days after conception, when the fetus is still only 1/20 of a inch long, this thickness becomes the neural groove. The groove closes over forming a tube, the forward end of which develops into the brain.

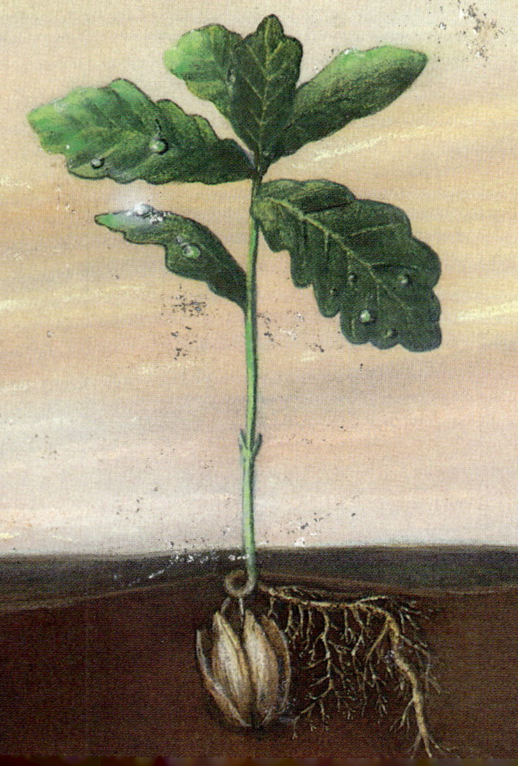

Building a Brain

The story of the human brain begins at the start of life itself. Only three weeks after the first cell division of conception, a tiny sheet of cells appears on the back of the minute embryo and grows at a feverish rate, creating millions of new brain cells each day. From this moment until death, the brain will undergo constant change as its 14 billion nerve cells, called neurons, first create the increasingly complex interconnections that typify the healthy, adult brain, then start to die off and lose some of those vital connections as they age.

During gestation, the brain grows into a two-thirds-sized likeness of its adult self. At birth its anatomy is virtually complete. The rumpled cortex, that familiar outer layer that gives the brain its walnut-like appearance, covers the inner structures protectively, just as it does in an adult brain. But there is still work to be done. Every neuron must set out to make connections with others of its kind. And each cell must be wrapped in its own insulating material. These branching connectors and the insulating sheaths are responsible for the increasing weight and size of the brain in the growing child. The cells of the cortex move apart and thus create enough room for the extra weight and volume of the maturing brain.

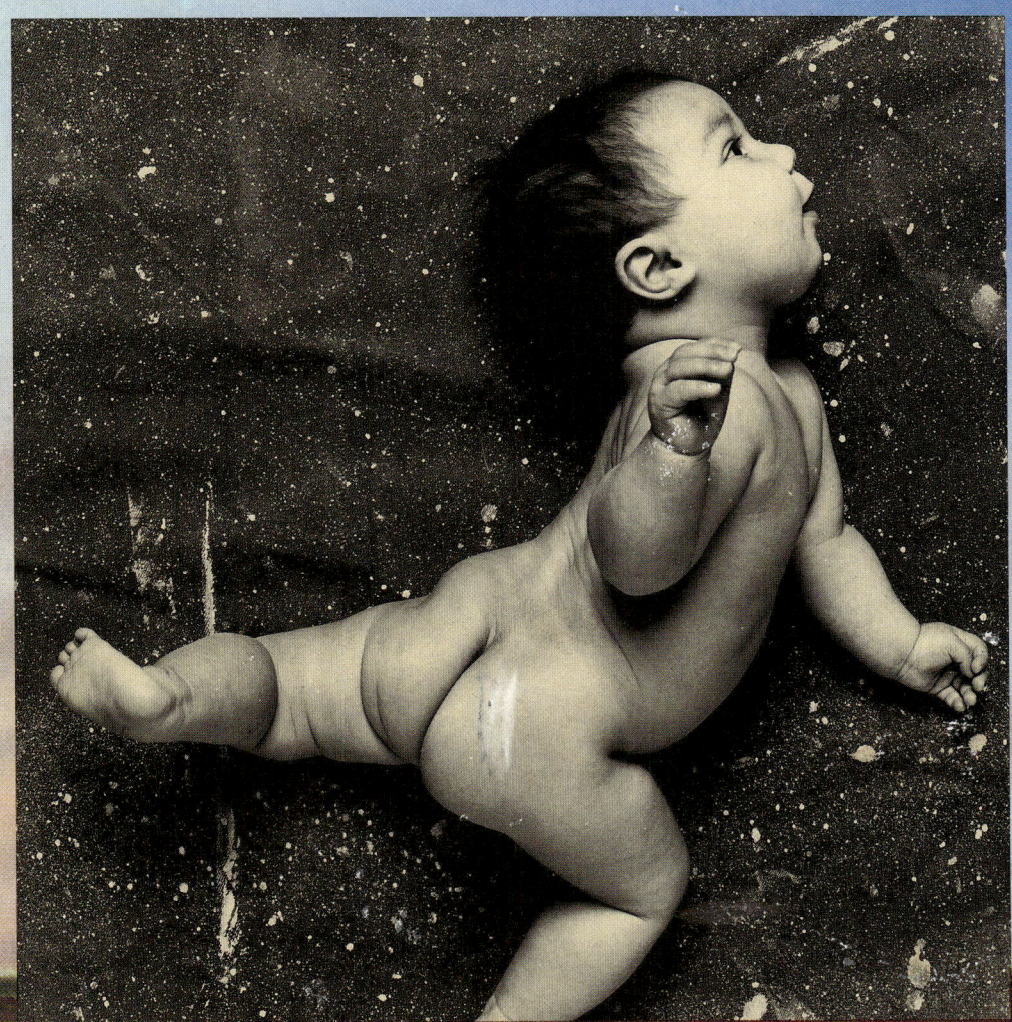

Babies are born with very nearly a full complement of 14 billion neurons in their brains. A few more neurons may form in the first months after birth, but from then on no more are produced.

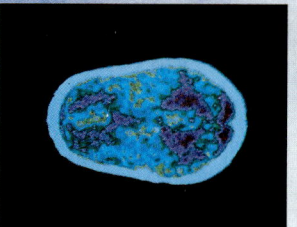 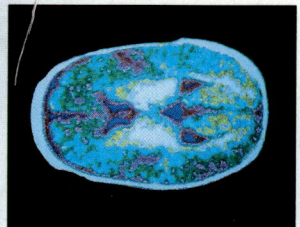 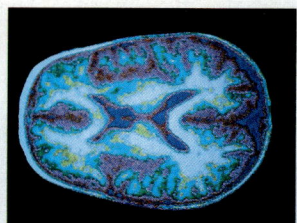 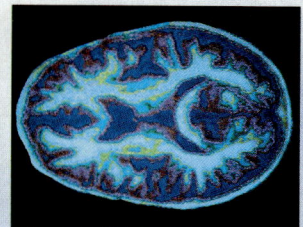

Magnetic resonance imaging (MRI) scans show the developing tissue of the human brain. In a newborn (scan at far left) the brain weighs about a tenth of its eventual 1,300 to 1,500 grams, making it the human organ closest to adult size at birth. The brain is also 10 percent of body weight at birth. By six months (second scan), the baby's brain will be half its adult weight. At 20 months (third scan) weight and size have increased again because of the rapid growth of supporting cells, called glia, which grow after birth. At 9 to 10 years (fourth scan) the head and brain are at virtually full adult size—about 2 percent of body weight.

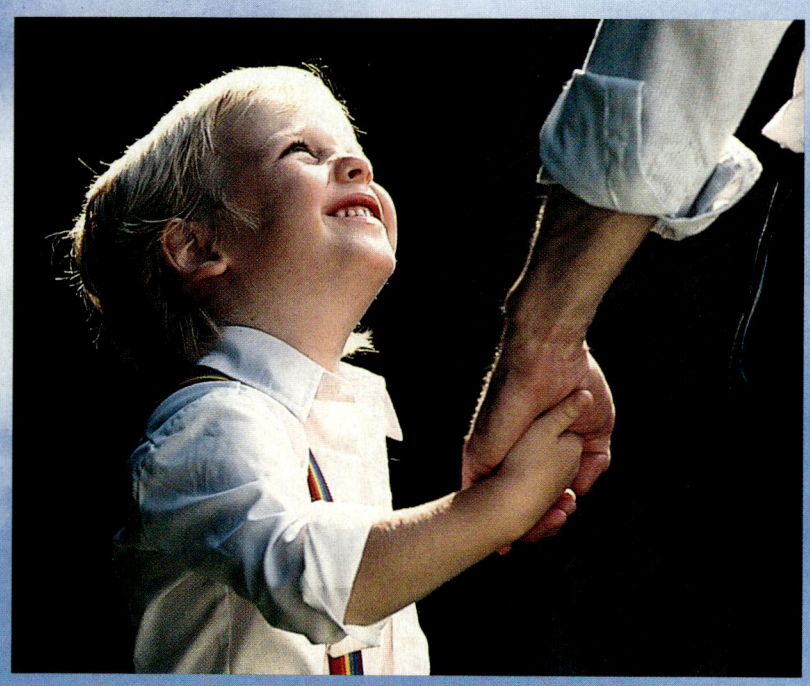

Within four years, the brain has masterminded a host of incredibly complex processes to produce a walking, talking, thinking, feeling, reasoning being.

Nerve cells such as these are virtually all in place by birth. However an insulating sheath, called myelin, grows around parts of the each nerve cell after birth. This insulation ensures smooth transmission of the messages sent by neurons.

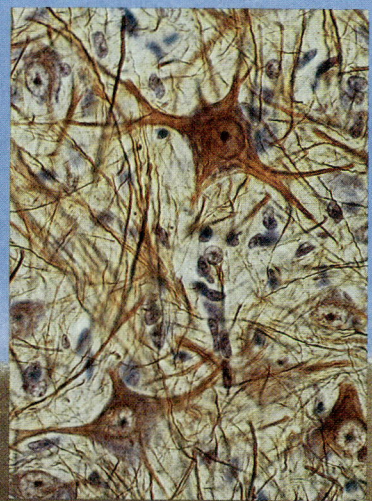

BUILDING A BRAIN

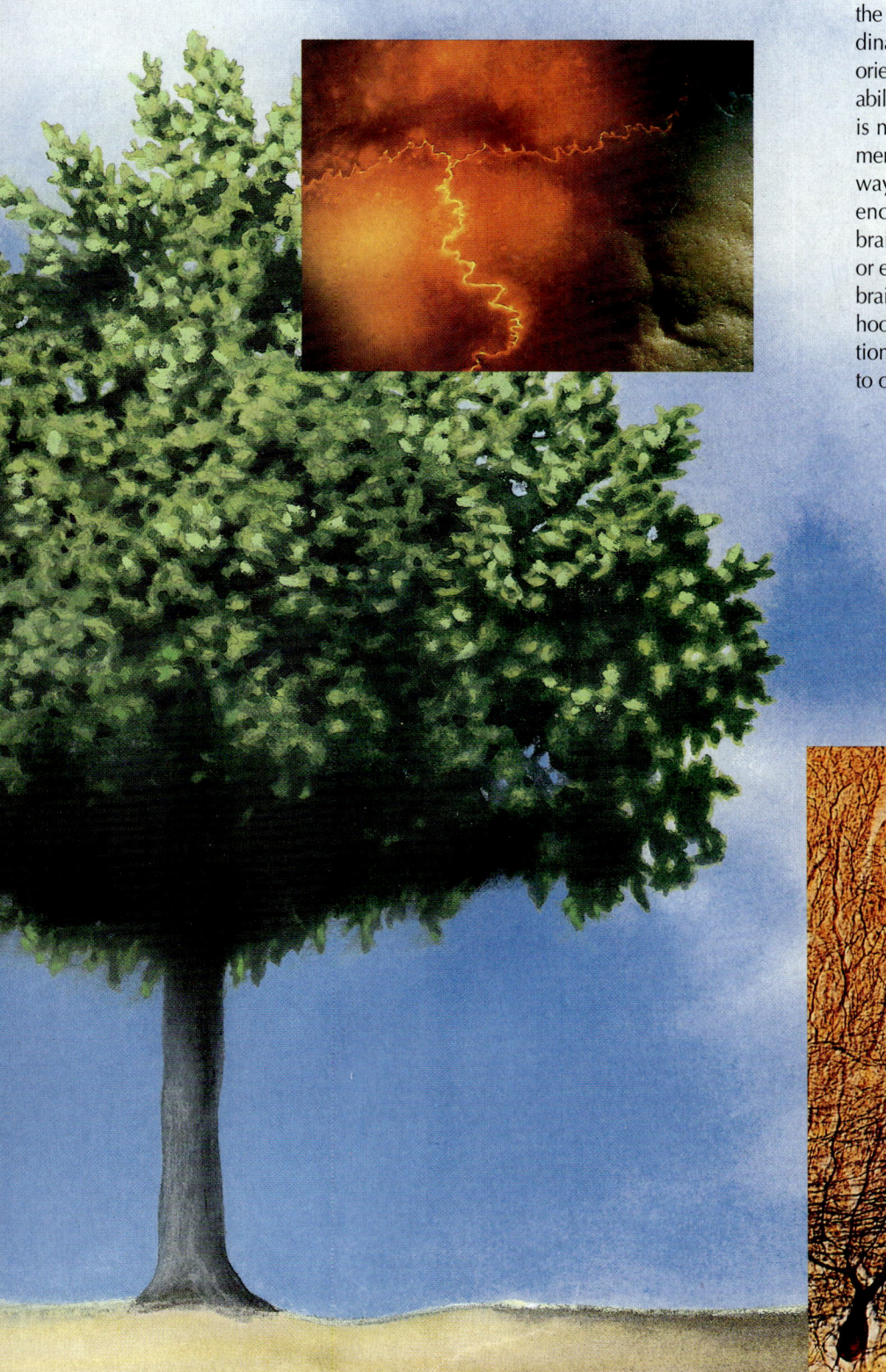

The housing for the human brain consists of eight thin, interlocking, domed plates. These cranial bones are not yet fully grown, nor are they joined at birth; the plates are squeezed and overlap during passage through the birth canal. Fusion will be complete by about 18 months.

Neural connections become increasingly more complicated as the brain matures. In the cortex alone each cell is estimated to have as many as 10,000 connections, making the number of possible connections in one human cortex about 200,000 times the population of Earth. Everything rests on the precision of these contacts—motor coordination, perception, the retention of memories, the acquisition of a vocabulary and the ability to develop patterns of thought. But this is not a passive process. External environment and stimuli cause many of these pathways to be forged. Genes and outside influences act together to create each unique brain, and deprivation of any sort—sensory or emotional—can distort the growth of the brain. The brain-building processes of childhood form the basis for the refined perception and exquisite motor control necessary to operate in the adult world.

Neurons from the human brain show the complex network of interconnection that develops after birth. The increasing connections are responsible for the growth in brain size after birth.

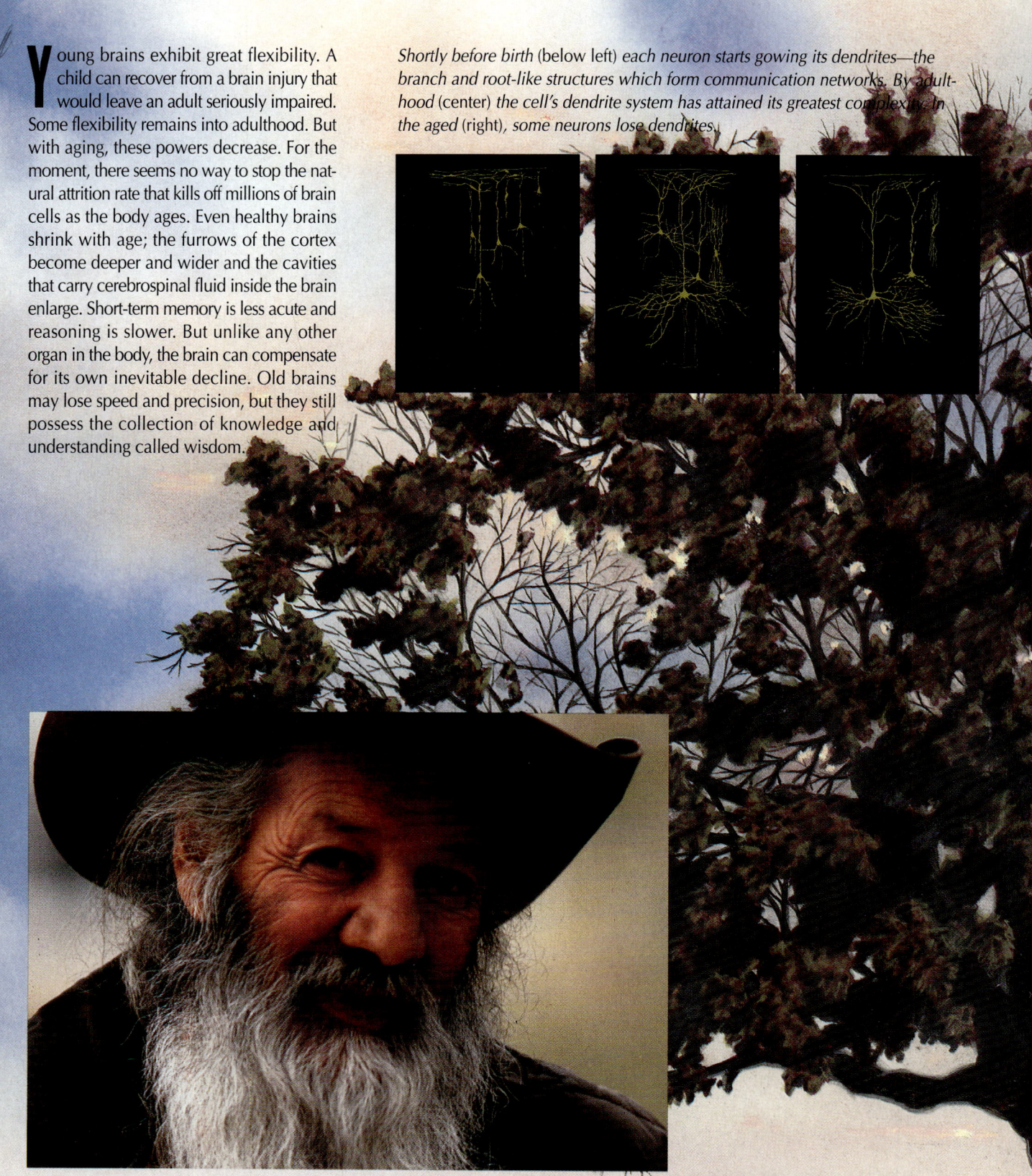

Young brains exhibit great flexibility. A child can recover from a brain injury that would leave an adult seriously impaired. Some flexibility remains into adulthood. But with aging, these powers decrease. For the moment, there seems no way to stop the natural attrition rate that kills off millions of brain cells as the body ages. Even healthy brains shrink with age; the furrows of the cortex become deeper and wider and the cavities that carry cerebrospinal fluid inside the brain enlarge. Short-term memory is less acute and reasoning is slower. But unlike any other organ in the body, the brain can compensate for its own inevitable decline. Old brains may lose speed and precision, but they still possess the collection of knowledge and understanding called wisdom.

Shortly before birth (below left) *each neuron starts gowing its dendrites—the branch and root-like structures which form communication networks. By adulthood* (center) *the cell's dendrite system has attained its greatest complexity. In the aged* (right), *some neurons lose dendrites.*

In a healthy elderly person, some neurons may actually increase their connecting dendrites in an effort to make up for those that have been lost in natural aging.

BUILDING A BRAIN

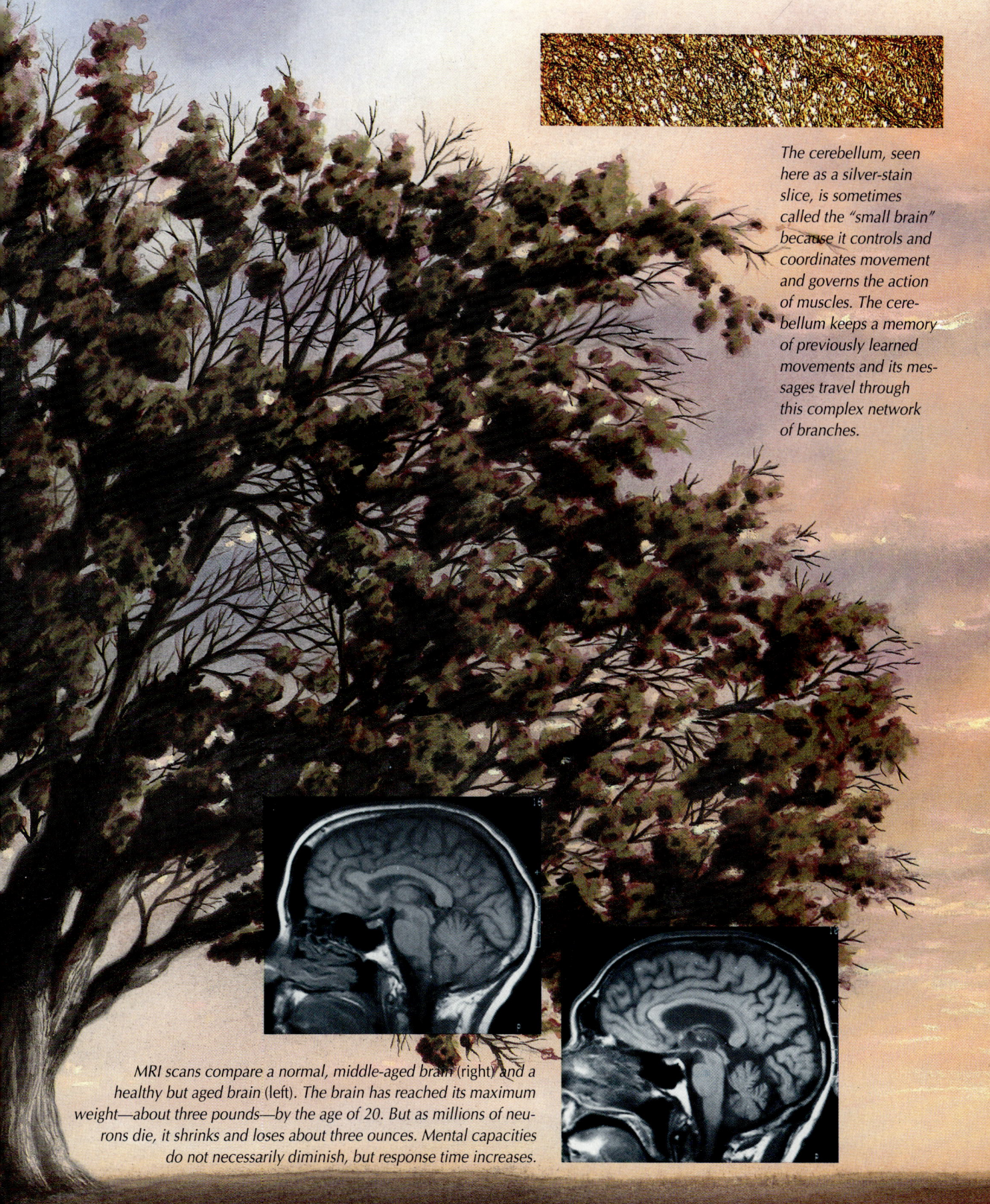

The cerebellum, seen here as a silver-stain slice, is sometimes called the "small brain" because it controls and coordinates movement and governs the action of muscles. The cerebellum keeps a memory of previously learned movements and its messages travel through this complex network of branches.

MRI scans compare a normal, middle-aged brain (right) and a healthy but aged brain (left). The brain has reached its maximum weight—about three pounds—by the age of 20. But as millions of neurons die, it shrinks and loses about three ounces. Mental capacities do not necessarily diminish, but response time increases.

STAYING ALIVE

The human brain. Perhaps alone in all of nature, it is the only organ that is aware of itself, aware of the universe that surrounds it, aware of life and death. It has been described—with understatement—as the world's most complex structure. It is more than a living computer: It empowers humans with the capacities to create poetry and music, sculpture and machinery, to think, to speak and to love. For thousands of years, even such great thinkers as the Greek philosopher Aristotle regarded the heart as the seat of thought and senses. But in the last century, neuroscientists have made extraordinary progress in penetrating the physical mysteries of the brain. Now the convoluted, three-pound mass of pinkish-gray tissue that Aristotle believed served only to cool the blood is unveiled as a network of some 14 billion nerve cells, coordinating not only thought and the senses, but most bodily activity as well. Using microscopes and X-rays, surgical skills and electrodes, scientists have discerned that brain activity depends on coordinated chemical reactions and electrochemical energy equivalent to that required to light a 10-watt bulb.

They know that the brain, comprised of many cooperative subsystems, is more of an organization than an organ. They understand that the brain and spinal cord choreograph conscious physical movement, that the brain is the body's internal caretaker, continually monitoring its well-being so that human beings breathe, circulate blood, fight infections, sleep and wake, reproduce, eat and digest foods at rates that preserve general health throughout a lifetime.

And they can state that the brain makes possible not only logic and abstract thought, but also sensory awareness, language, creativity, memory and the capacity for altruism, confirming what Hippocrates, the Greek father of medicine, guessed 2,400 years ago: "From the brain and from the brain only arise our pleasures, joys, laughter, and jests as well as our sorrows, pains, griefs, and fears."

But after the sum of all these functions is taken, it still is difficult to appreciate fully the wondrous complexity of the human brain. How is it that this collection

---

Interwoven in dense networks, nerve cells—or neurons—work round the clock, relaying split-second electrochemical messages, most of which concern the brain's primary responsibility: keeping the body alive.

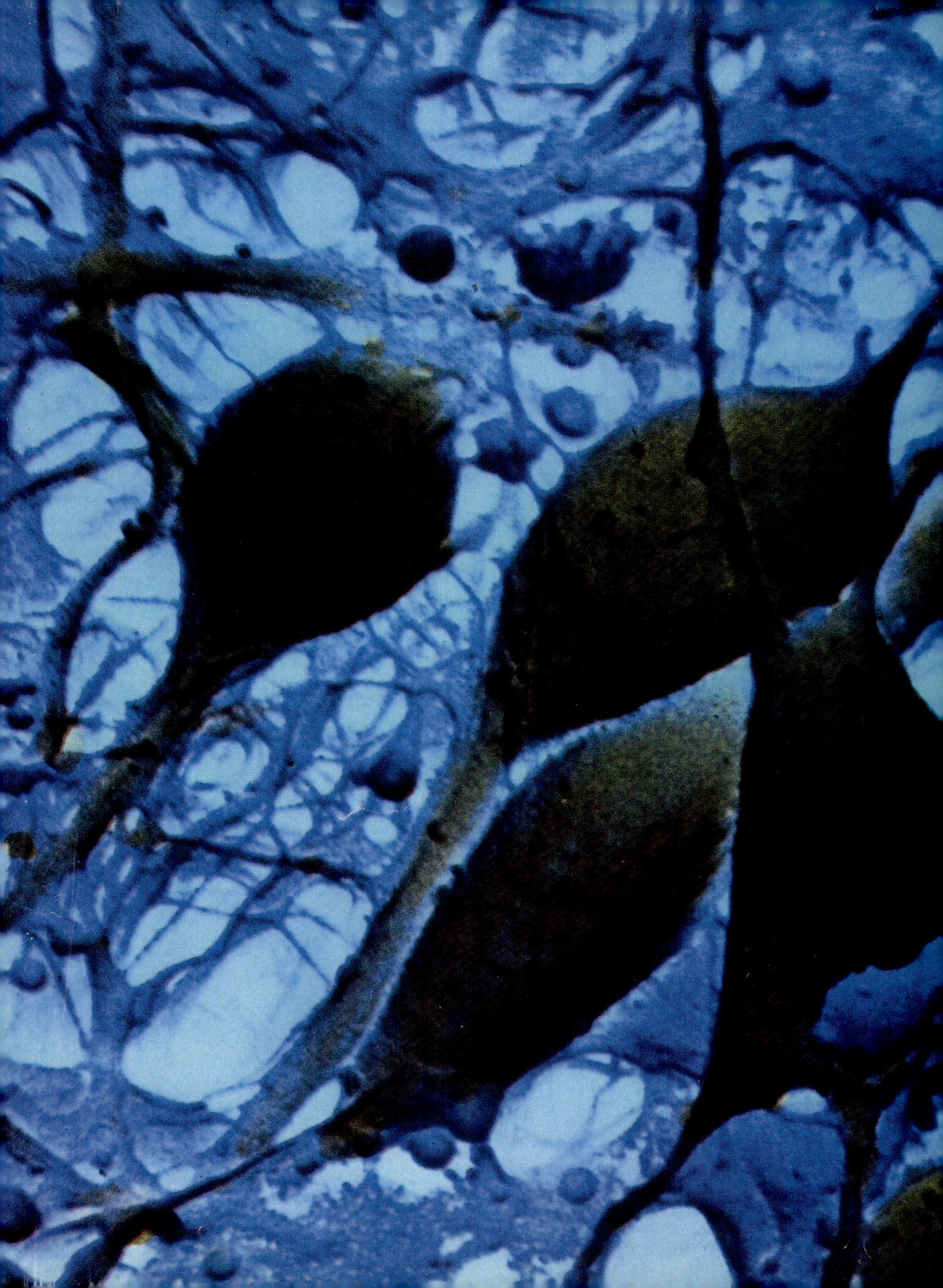

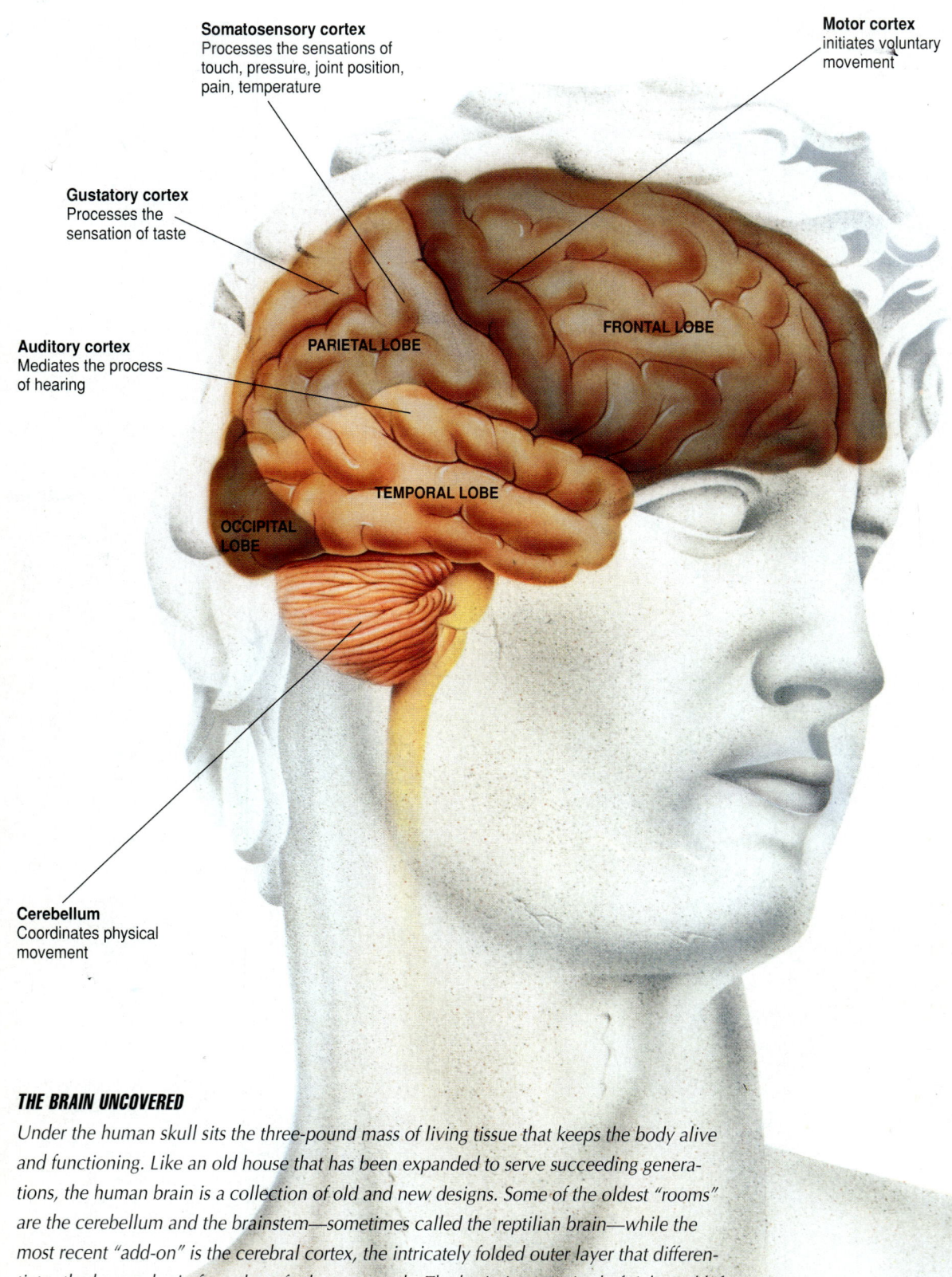

THE BRAIN UNCOVERED

Under the human skull sits the three-pound mass of living tissue that keeps the body alive and functioning. Like an old house that has been expanded to serve succeeding generations, the human brain is a collection of old and new designs. Some of the oldest "rooms" are the cerebellum and the brainstem—sometimes called the reptilian brain—while the most recent "add-on" is the cerebral cortex, the intricately folded outer layer that differentiates the human brain from that of other mammals. The brain is comprised of right and left halves, or hemispheres, each of which has four lobes where information is received and analyzed and from which messages are sent to various parts of the body.

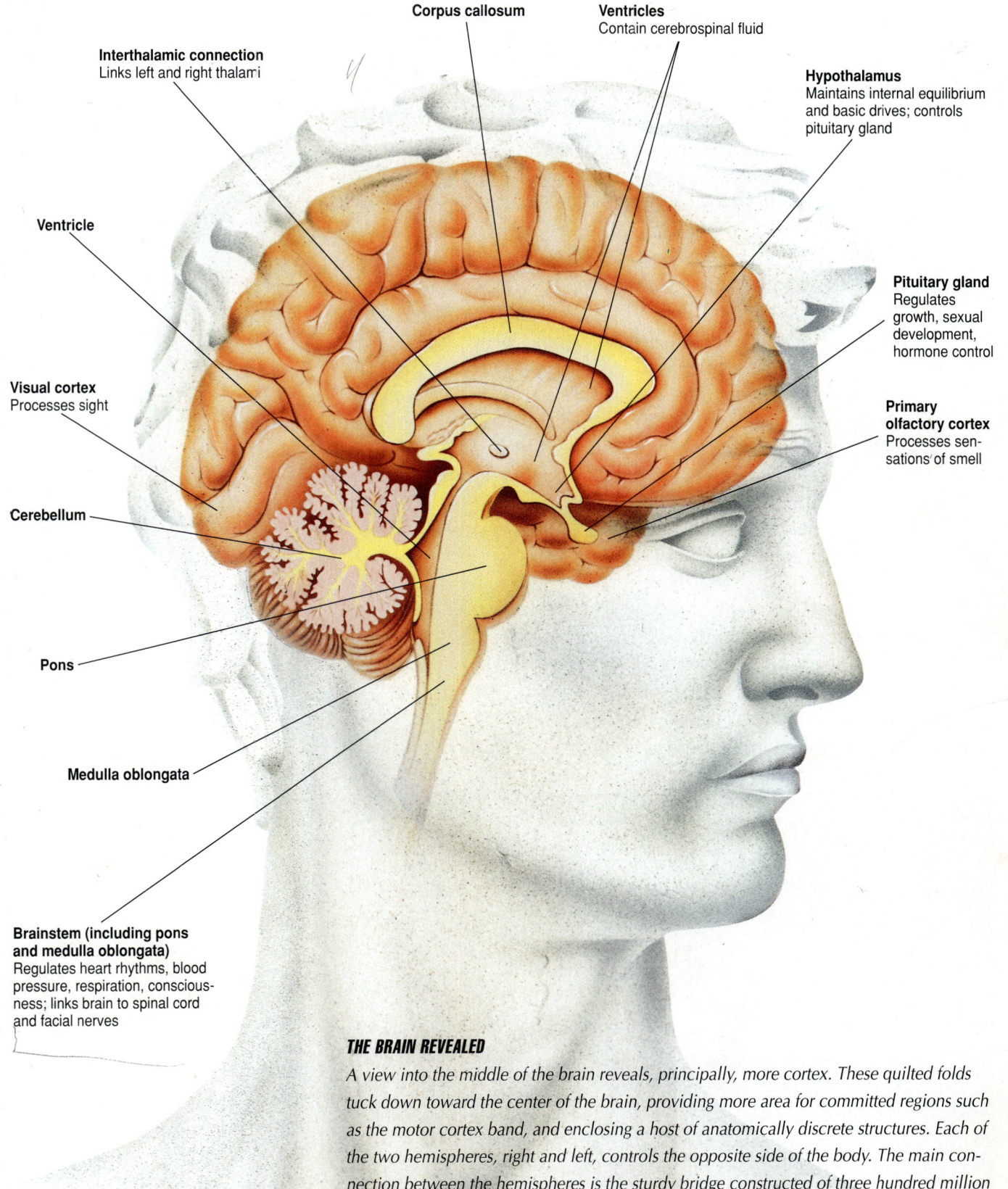

Corpus callosum

Ventricles
Contain cerebrospinal fluid

Interthalamic connection
Links left and right thalami

Hypothalamus
Maintains internal equilibrium and basic drives; controls pituitary gland

Ventricle

Pituitary gland
Regulates growth, sexual development, hormone control

Visual cortex
Processes sight

Primary olfactory cortex
Processes sensations of smell

Cerebellum

Pons

Medulla oblongata

Brainstem (including pons and medulla oblongata)
Regulates heart rhythms, blood pressure, respiration, consciousness; links brain to spinal cord and facial nerves

THE BRAIN REVEALED

A view into the middle of the brain reveals, principally, more cortex. These quilted folds tuck down toward the center of the brain, providing more area for committed regions such as the motor cortex band, and enclosing a host of anatomically discrete structures. Each of the two hemispheres, right and left, controls the opposite side of the body. The main connection between the hemispheres is the sturdy bridge constructed of three hundred million nerve fibers known as the corpus callosum. Though each hemisphere seems to have specific areas of responsibility, the corpus callosum is their communication link and passes information from one side to the other.

of living tissues creates in each human being something beyond examination, so full of unique memories, dreams, plans and desires as to be quite unlike any other.

RUNNING THE MACHINE

Any understanding of the brain begins with its smallest working units—the nerve cells, or neurons, that form a complex network to direct the body's every move and thought. Neurons, all 14 billion of them, are distinguished by their specialized ability to receive and transmit electrochemical signals either from inside the body—fever or stomach pain, for example—or from the outside world—a voice or a pinprick. Depending on their location, these neurons may respond to information through reflexive or voluntary movement, memory, thought, judgment or emotional behavior.

Forming a supportive framework for the neural network are the glial cells. Glia provide a kind of matrix in which the neurons of the embryonic brain grow and mature. There are from five to ten times as many glial cells as neurons and they come in a number of varieties. One type forms myelin, an insulating material that wraps around parts of the neurons; another bridges nerve cells and blood vessels, delivering nourishment to the neurons and removing their waste products. These cells, named astrocytes for their star shape, play a part in the so-called blood-brain barrier, a shield protecting the capillaries in the brain. Like gatekeepers, astrocytes monitor and selectively admit certain substances through the tight junctions of brain capillaries.

The neurons themselves resemble tree trunks growing from a frizzle of roots—a design that enables them to courier messages to any point in the body in microseconds. Most of the roots, called dendrites, are relatively short and are built principally to receive incoming messages from other neurons. The trunk-like axon is engineered to transmit messages to other neurons. While axons can be as short as a few millionths of an inch—in the brain—they can be as long as a yard—the

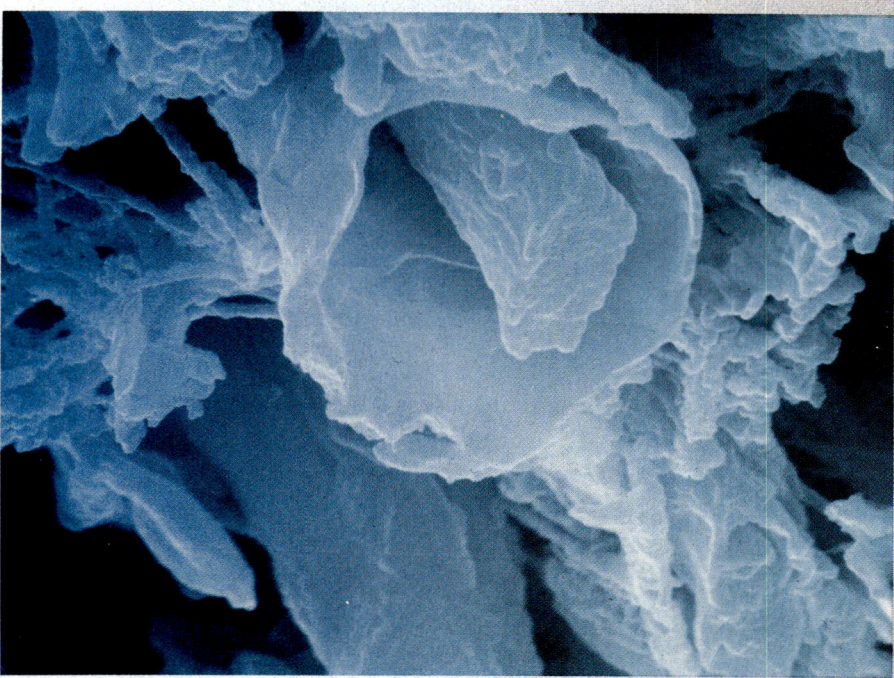

Capillary
Capillaries transport blood to the brain, a glutton for oxygen and glucose. 25 percent of the blood pumped by each heartbeat goes to the brain.

COURIERS OF THE BRAIN
The basic working unit of the brain is the nerve cell, or neuron, (right). The axon at left has a degenerated myelin sheath, characteristic of multiple sclerosis. As the insulating myelin deteriorates, the consequent disrupted communication results in neural and muscular dysfunctions.

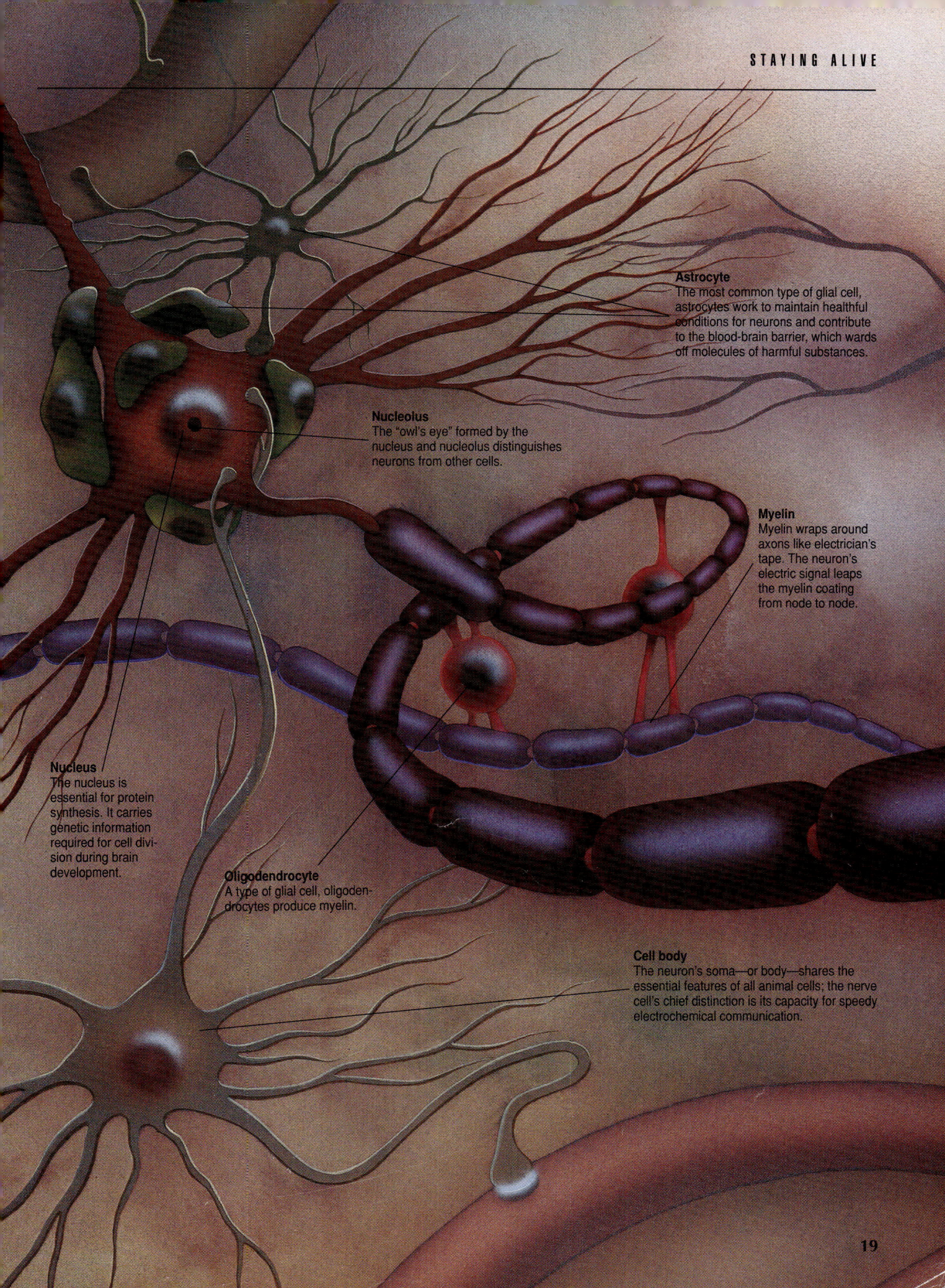

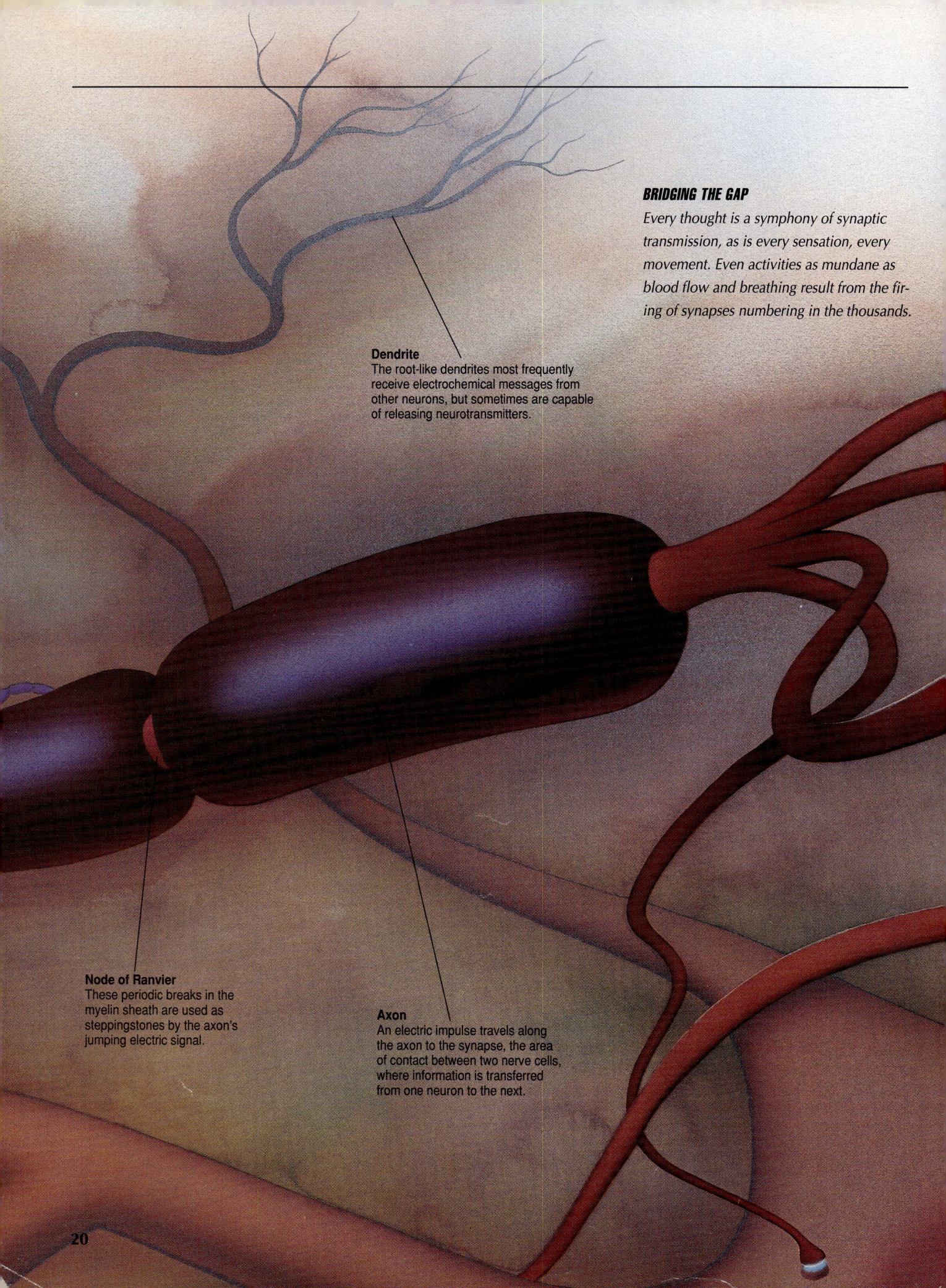

BRIDGING THE GAP
Every thought is a symphony of synaptic transmission, as is every sensation, every movement. Even activities as mundane as blood flow and breathing result from the firing of synapses numbering in the thousands.

Dendrite
The root-like dendrites most frequently receive electrochemical messages from other neurons, but sometimes are capable of releasing neurotransmitters.

Node of Ranvier
These periodic breaks in the myelin sheath are used as steppingstones by the axon's jumping electric signal.

Axon
An electric impulse travels along the axon to the synapse, the area of contact between two nerve cells, where information is transferred from one neuron to the next.

sciatic nerve of a tall adult. Most axons are sheathed in the myelin that acts both to preserve the electrochemical signals and speed their transmission. Some myelinated neurons can transmit at a rate of 120 miles per hour. (The lack of muscular finesse in infants results, in part, from short-circuited signals crossing axons that have not yet been myelinated.)

Neurons owe their electrochemical properties to a dynamic imbalance of charged chemical particles, called ions, between the inside and outside of each cell. The communication system goes to work when a neurotransmitter, the potent chemical courier that travels from one neuron to another, stimulates receptors on the surface of a dendrite. Activation of the receptor then initiates a chain of chemical events within the neuron, resulting in an influx of positively charged ions from outside the cell. This, in turn, triggers an electrical discharge that then, like a burning fuse, follows the trunk-like axon to its terminal. There, at the tip of the terminal, tiny sacs release minute quantities of a particular neurotransmitter—dozens of different types have been identified—into the gap at the end of the terminal. The presence of a neurotransmitter in this gap, called the synaptic cleft, is detected

Synaptic vesicles
These tiny sacs release their cargo of neurotransmitters into the synaptic cleft.

Presynaptic terminal
Having traveled the length of the axon, the electric signal triggers neurotransmitter release at the axon's terminal.

Synaptic cleft
The gap between neurons where a message, converted from electric to chemical energy, crosses to the post-synaptic neuron.

Receptor site
The neurotransmitter binds to a specialized receptor on the post-synaptic neuron. One receptor site may have receptors for several neurotransmitter types.

by receptors on a receiving neuron and the electrochemical reaction begins anew as the message is passed to its final destination.

At the same time, the first neuron, having discharged its neurotransmitter, undergoes a brief recovery period, measured in thousandths of a second, after which it is ready to fire again. Given the fact that any one neuron may form 5,000 to 50,000 connections with its neighbors, the number of possible synapses in the brain outnumbers the stars in the Milky Way a hundredfold.

Despite the overwhelming number of neurons, their growth and distribution is no haphazard arrangement. Rather, groups of similarly functioning cells cluster together in discrete masses called nuclei (when they are associated with the brain and spinal cord), or ganglia (when they are found elsewhere in the body). Some of these clusters act as relay stations along the "hard-wired" neural pathways that keep the senses, skele-tal muscles and visceral organs operating. But in the brain the vast majority of neurons, as many as 97 percent, are so-called interneurons, involved in what neuroscientists refer to as "association" tasks.

Interneurons are uncommitted at the time of a baby's birth; their synaptic pathways are up for grabs. Over time and as the result of events and learning, repetition and experience, they weave synaptic cross-links with the warp of countless programmed pathways in other parts of the brain. Simply stated, this is what allows the growing child to know and do more with every passing month. And it is the interneurons that make it possible to associate a familiar face with a familiar voice, and then to reach into the mental data bank for emotional reactions a fraction of a second later.

Based on their location, neurons are further classified as belonging to either the central or peripheral nervous systems, the body's two control networks. The central nervous system (CNS)—the command center—is comprised of the two-hemisphered brain and the spinal cord, the main trunk line to outlying districts. The CNS receives sensory data, makes conscious and unconscious decisions based on the information, and responds with appropriate commands, often carried out by the peripheral nervous system (PNS). When light is shone into the eyes, for example, nuclei in the brainstem dispatch a command—through the peripheral nervous system—to constrict the iris.

The peripheral nervous system consists of 40-odd pairs of nerves, with some cells originating in the spinal cord. Most of the nerves on the left side of the body cross over to communicate with the right hemisphere of the brain; their counterparts on the right side of the body link up with the brain's left hemisphere. Nerve fibers belonging to the PNS are further classified according to function as being somatic (bodily) or autonomic (self-regulating). Somatic nerves are responsible for sensory awareness, as well as muscular actions that are either voluntary or reflexive. Autonomic nerves are dedicated to the unconscious regulation

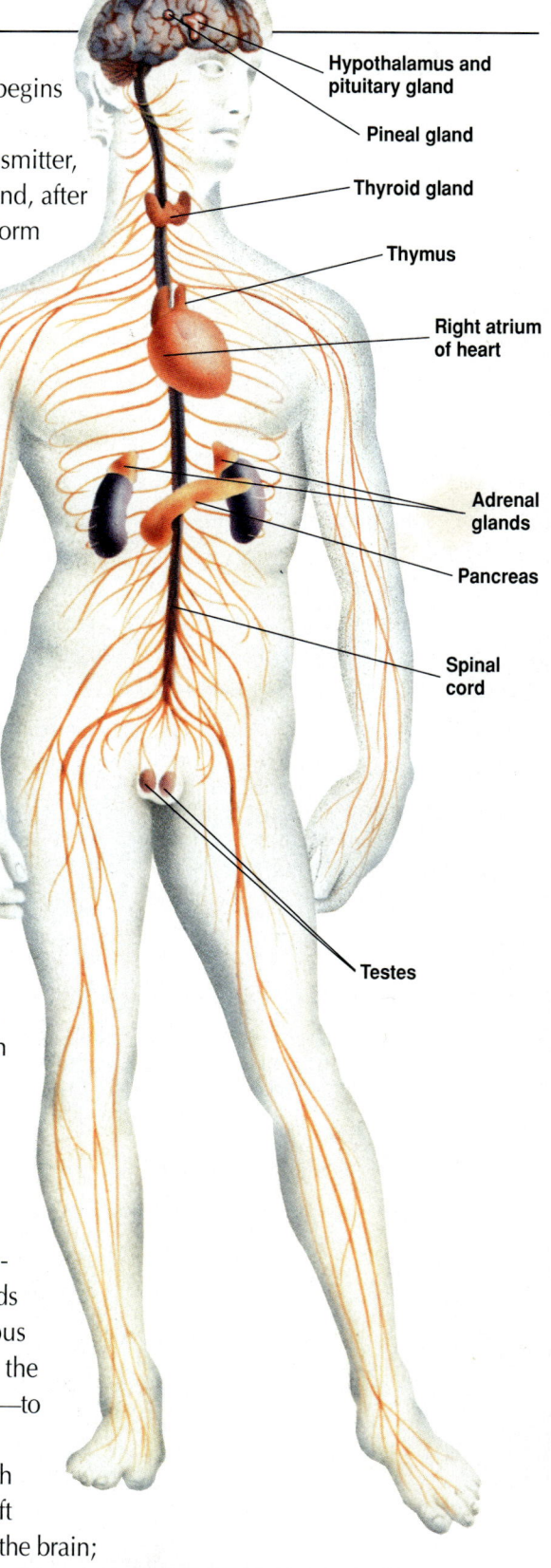

THE NEUROENDOCRINE SYSTEM
The glands of the endocrine system (labeled above) work in conjunction with the two sub-systems of the nervous system: central *(brain and spinal cord) and peripheral.*

of such things as heartbeat, skin temperature and perspiration. Together, the somatic and autonomic subsystems extend the reach of the brain's influence and awareness to every corner of the body.

Both subsystems manage multiple roles by means of a two-way communications line. A feedback loop, working much like a thermostat, relays body information to the central nervous system, where an assessment is made and a corrective order sent to the relevant organ. In the somatic system, for example, a chain of motor nerves descends from the brain and spinal cord and fans out to skeletal muscles, directing every kind of movement from the reflexive blink of an eyelid to the conscious tapping of a toe. Sensory nerves transmit in the opposite direction, their impulses entering the spinal cord and brain on an ascending pathway to deliver information about the skin, joints, muscles and sensory organs.

In most instances the information is not urgent, and the brain has time to make the decision to move a hand or foot voluntarily. But if the information is critical—a hand touching a hot stove, for instance—the system shortcuts the brain alarm at the spinal cord, to initiate almost instantaneous reflex action.

In spinal reflexes the entire event from stimulus to response may involve just one sensory neuron's communication to one motor neuron, as in the classic knee-jerk reaction, but more likely the circuit passes through at least one interneuron. More complex adjustments—such as the shifting of body weight to maintain bal-

HYPOTHALAMUS AND PITUITARY GLAND
This team, consisting of two of the most influential structures in the brain, controls essential bodily functions. Many commands originating in the hypothalamus travel by neurotransmission to other areas of the nervous system; those involving endocrine glands are regulated by the pituitary and sent through the bloodstream.

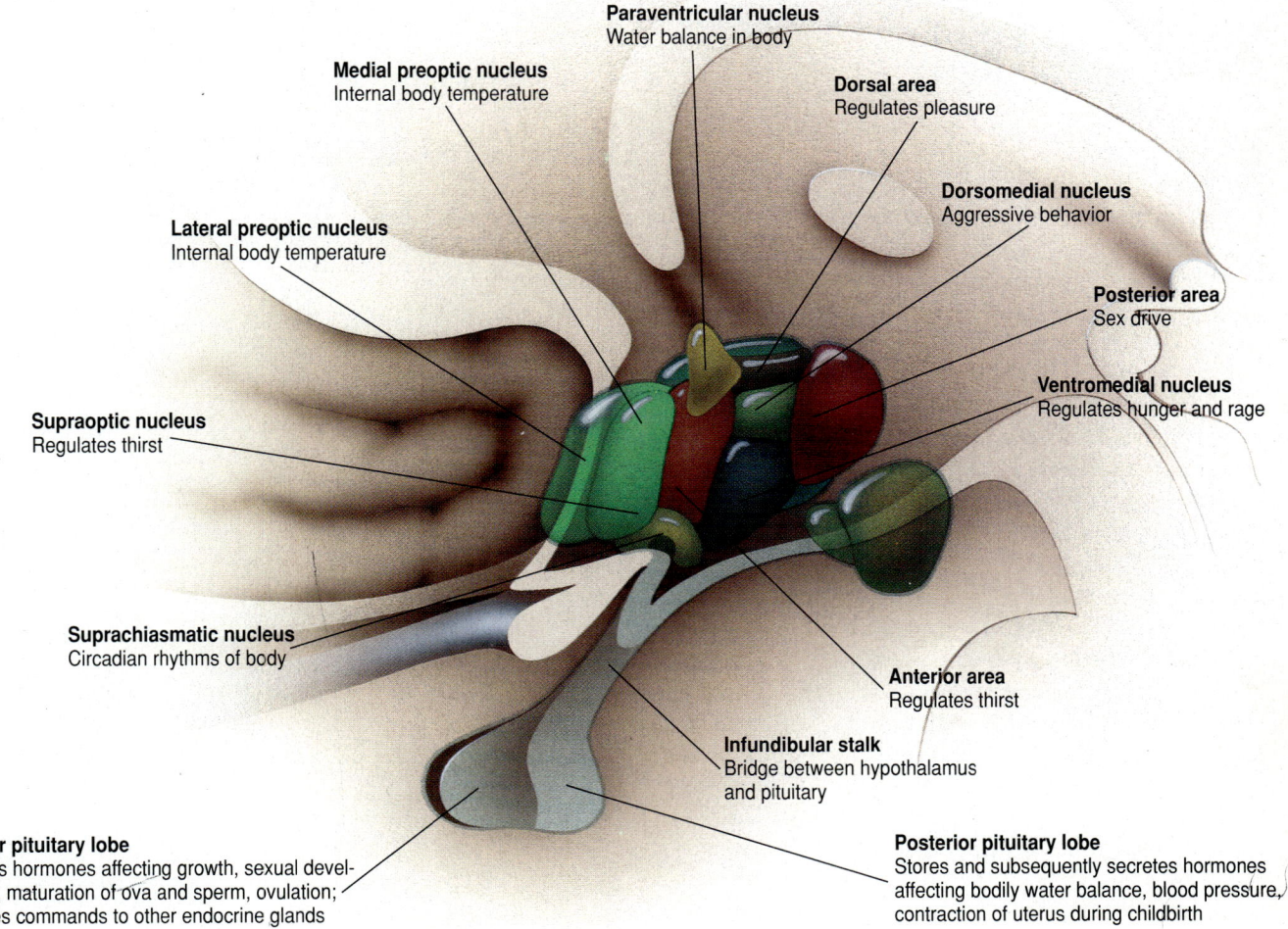

Paraventricular nucleus
Water balance in body

Medial preoptic nucleus
Internal body temperature

Dorsal area
Regulates pleasure

Dorsomedial nucleus
Aggressive behavior

Lateral preoptic nucleus
Internal body temperature

Posterior area
Sex drive

Ventromedial nucleus
Regulates hunger and rage

Supraoptic nucleus
Regulates thirst

Suprachiasmatic nucleus
Circadian rhythms of body

Anterior area
Regulates thirst

Infundibular stalk
Bridge between hypothalamus and pituitary

Anterior pituitary lobe
Secretes hormones affecting growth, sexual development, maturation of ova and sperm, ovulation; regulates commands to other endocrine glands

Posterior pituitary lobe
Stores and subsequently secretes hormones affecting bodily water balance, blood pressure, contraction of uterus during childbirth

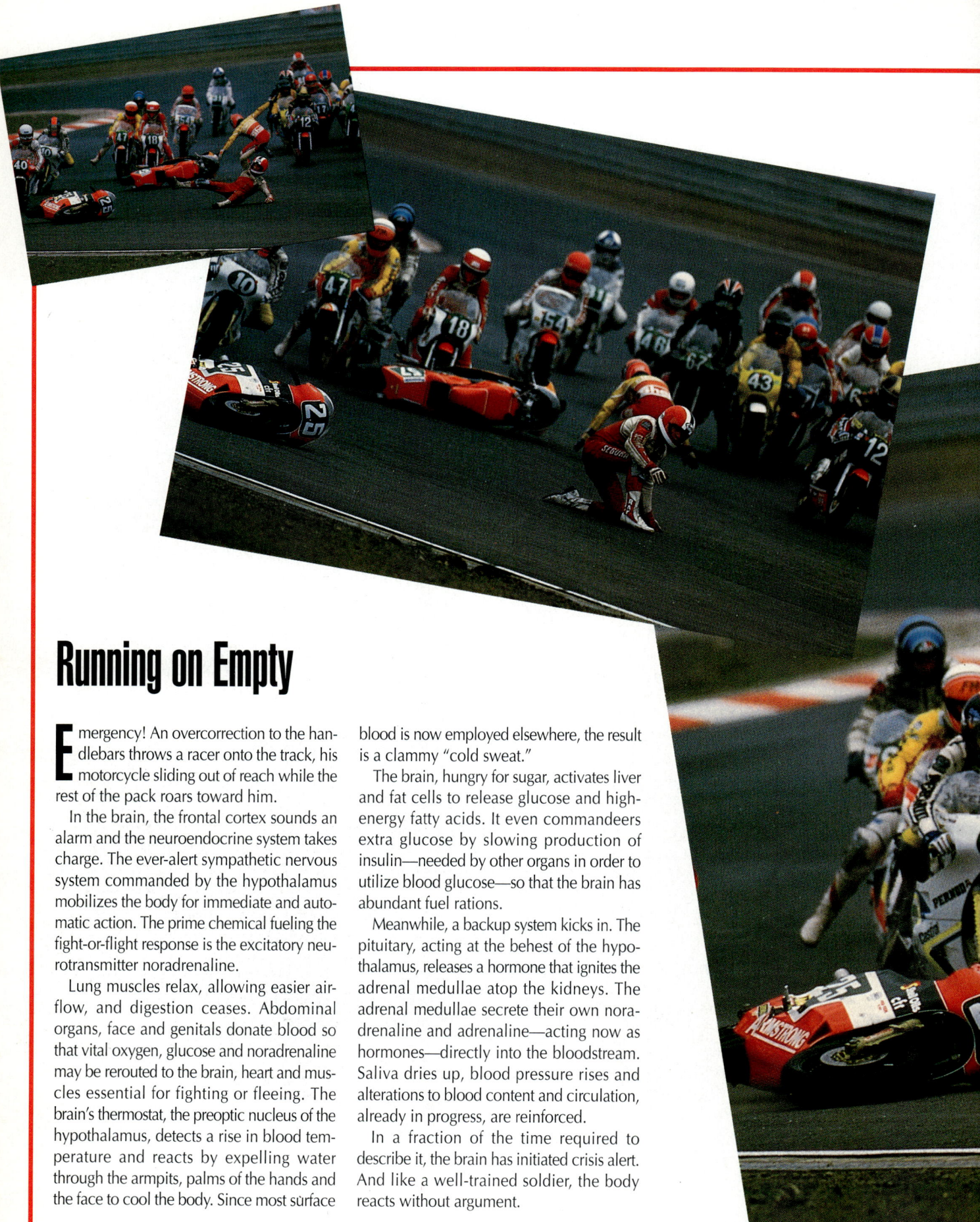

Running on Empty

Emergency! An overcorrection to the handlebars throws a racer onto the track, his motorcycle sliding out of reach while the rest of the pack roars toward him.

In the brain, the frontal cortex sounds an alarm and the neuroendocrine system takes charge. The ever-alert sympathetic nervous system commanded by the hypothalamus mobilizes the body for immediate and automatic action. The prime chemical fueling the fight-or-flight response is the excitatory neurotransmitter noradrenaline.

Lung muscles relax, allowing easier airflow, and digestion ceases. Abdominal organs, face and genitals donate blood so that vital oxygen, glucose and noradrenaline may be rerouted to the brain, heart and muscles essential for fighting or fleeing. The brain's thermostat, the preoptic nucleus of the hypothalamus, detects a rise in blood temperature and reacts by expelling water through the armpits, palms of the hands and the face to cool the body. Since most surface blood is now employed elsewhere, the result is a clammy "cold sweat."

The brain, hungry for sugar, activates liver and fat cells to release glucose and high-energy fatty acids. It even commandeers extra glucose by slowing production of insulin—needed by other organs in order to utilize blood glucose—so that the brain has abundant fuel rations.

Meanwhile, a backup system kicks in. The pituitary, acting at the behest of the hypothalamus, releases a hormone that ignites the adrenal medullae atop the kidneys. The adrenal medullae secrete their own noradrenaline and adrenaline—acting now as hormones—directly into the bloodstream. Saliva dries up, blood pressure rises and alterations to blood content and circulation, already in progress, are reinforced.

In a fraction of the time required to describe it, the brain has initiated crisis alert. And like a well-trained soldier, the body reacts without argument.

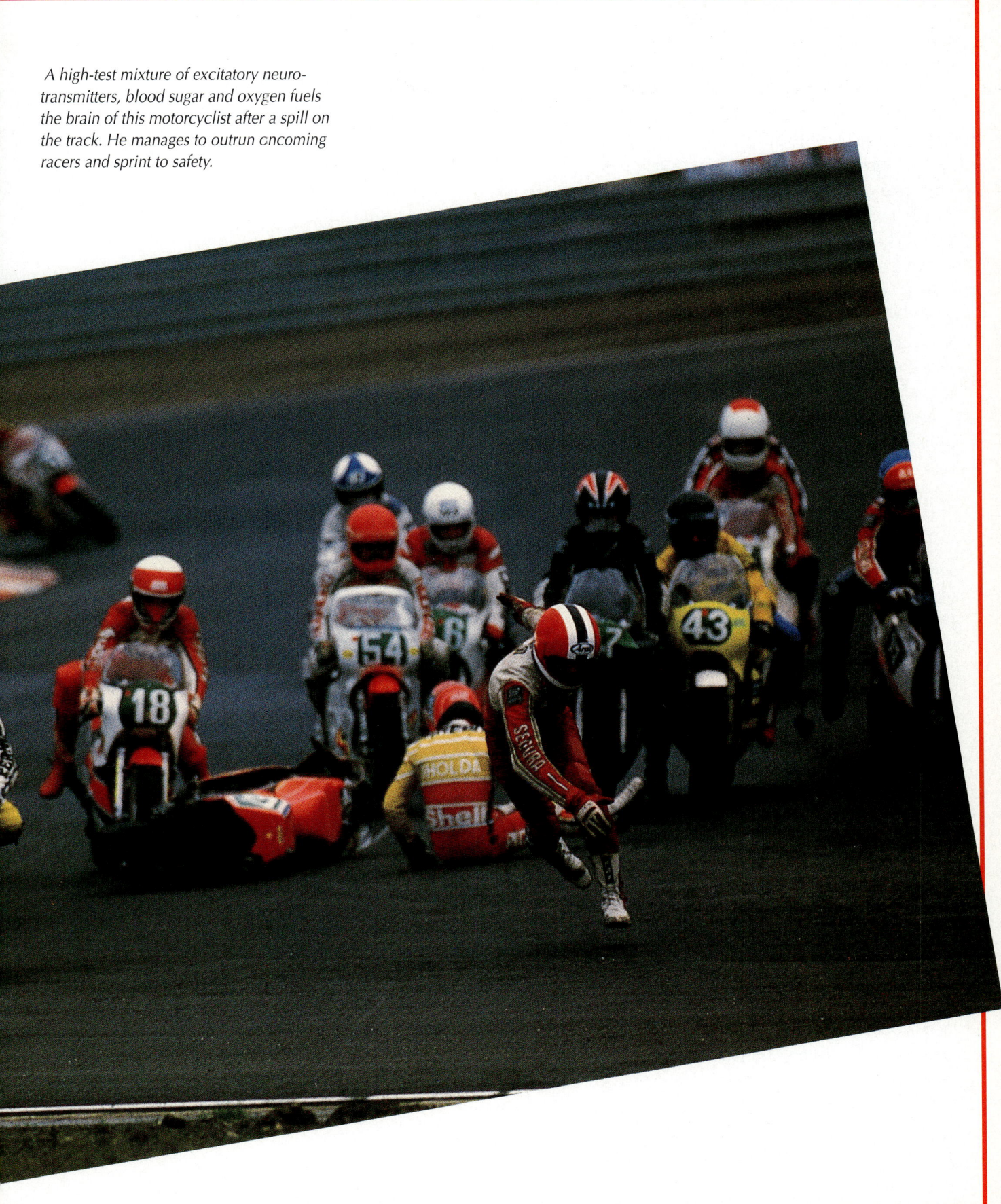

A high-test mixture of excitatory neurotransmitters, blood sugar and oxygen fuels the brain of this motorcyclist after a spill on the track. He manages to outrun oncoming racers and sprint to safety.

ance—may require hundreds of electrochemical messages involving both the spinal cord and the brain.

Like the involuntary aspects of somatic regulation, the autonomic subsystem is designed to work for the most part without conscious control. The autonomic system is dedicated to the activities of the heart, digestive system, lungs, reproductive organs, salivary and sweat glands, and the regulation of hunger, sleep, temperature and blood pressure. The purpose of the autonomic nervous system is to maintain a state of general equilibrium in the human body, and to help it respond to the relentless stimuli of the outside world. To do this, the system relies on two message tracts—sympathetic and parasympathetic. Sometimes these two systems oppose each other in much the same way as a car's gas and brake pedals accelerate and check speed. The sympathetic system speeds up the heart, for example, while the parasympathetic system slows it. In other situations the two cooperate to reach a common goal—the parasympathetic is responsible for male erection, while the sympathetic controls ejaculation.

A third autonomic division, the diffuse enteric nervous system, relies on the first two systems to help it regulate the digestive tract. At times, one of the two main systems will dominate—when the sympathetic system prepares the body for the fight or flight response, for example.

The limitation of dieting in regulating weight is a striking example of unconscious control over the body. The brain has certain setpoints—levels that are often genetically determined—to control appetite, the amount of digested food absorbed by the body and the rate at which calories are utilized as energy. Healthy eating restores the body's programmed weight, but will not alter it drastically from the brain's setting.

Generally it is the small but dynamic hypothalamus, along with its partner, the pituitary gland, that maintain bodily setpoints. While orders to most muscles are relayed cell-to-cell through the nervous system by neurotransmitters, instructions destined for endocrine glands travel through the blood as hormones released by the pituitary. The hypothalamus, both a gland and a neural structure, can secrete hormones as well as neurotransmitters. In its communication with the pituitary, the hypothalamus often uses direct neurotransmission, though it sometimes releases neurotransmitters into the bloodstream where they travel like hormones. The pituitary, as well as receiving commands from the hypothalamus, has its own work to do, which includes monitoring and regulating human growth.

Natural feedback mechanisms are not efficient enough for some highly reactive people. Known popularly as Type A people, their systems become so accustomed to running at top speed, constantly meeting real or imagined crises, that their setpoints adjust upward, leaving little or no time for the restorative mechanisms to work. Wear and tear on both body and emotions is the price paid.

The autonomic nervous system also has primary responsibility for a number of defense mechanisms designed to protect the body from disease—sneezing, shivering, fever, sweating and vomiting, for instance. More subtle but even more important to fighting infections and injuries is the immune system, which fights foreign

CUBE-CORNER CONUNDRUM

Staring at the center of this image presents the brain with a tough perceptual challenge: Is it a framed design of a protruding cube, or the inside corner of a wall? In fact it is both, but the brain, unsettled by ambiguity, clings first to one option and then the other. The result is a periodic visual flip-flop.

PATHWAYS OF VISION

Typical of many neural pathways, the fibers of the visual system transfer information from left to right and vice versa. Scientists do not know why much of the nervous system is arranged in this crisscross fashion.

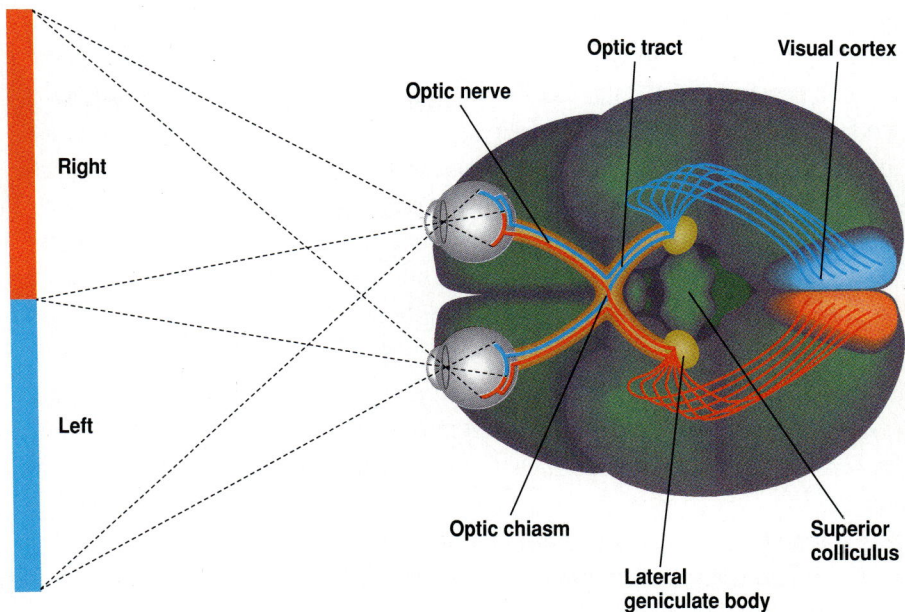

invaders through the production of antibodies. It has long been suspected that there is a link between an individual's susceptibility to infectious disease and his "state of mind." The favored theory is that prolonged stress impairs the vigorous functioning of the immune response. When the immune system is depressed, infection moves in with little resistance.

COMMON SENSES

Sensory systems come in many guises. Some—touch, pain and temperature—are experienced through sensory nerves scattered throughout the skin. Others—sight, hearing, smell and taste—are localized in unique organs. Still other mechanisms, including systems for monitoring blood pressure, blood sugar, thirst and fatigue, share certain characteristics of the classic senses.

As different as the messages may seem, all senses are similar in their basic action. Each relies on a well-coordinated team effort between several kinds of nerve cells, each communicates through the common language of electrochemical energy, and each is an afferent process (sending messages to the brain).

The common working units in virtually every sensory system are the sensory receptors; stalwart networks of them man the front lines of sensory experience. These receptors receive information from the outside world as they respond to the particular kind of energy to which they are sensitive—mechanical energy in the case of hearing and balance; chemical energy in taste and smell; radiant energy in sight. But the brain is equipped to trade only in the electrochemical energy of neurons. Each receptor cell, therefore, must operate as a transducer, or translator, converting the energy its dendrites receive into the usable electrochemical impulses that its axon can pass on.

As multiple receptor cells communicate with relay neurons farther along the line, they merge into larger nerve bundles and join a main trunk line. All sensations eventually pass through one of the thalami, the two major sensory integration centers, located roughly in the center of each hemisphere. These sensory messages are traveling to specialized regions of the cerebral cortex, in most cases their last stop in the processing journey. A latter stage of the processing of vision takes place at the back of the brain in the occipital, or visual, cortex. Sound is processed in the right and left halves of the primary auditory cortex, located near the ears within one of the deeper fissures of the enfolded cortex. The olfactory, or smell, pathway is the most eccentric, the odor trail leading first to two olfactory areas on the cortex, then to deeper, subcortical areas, including the thalamus.

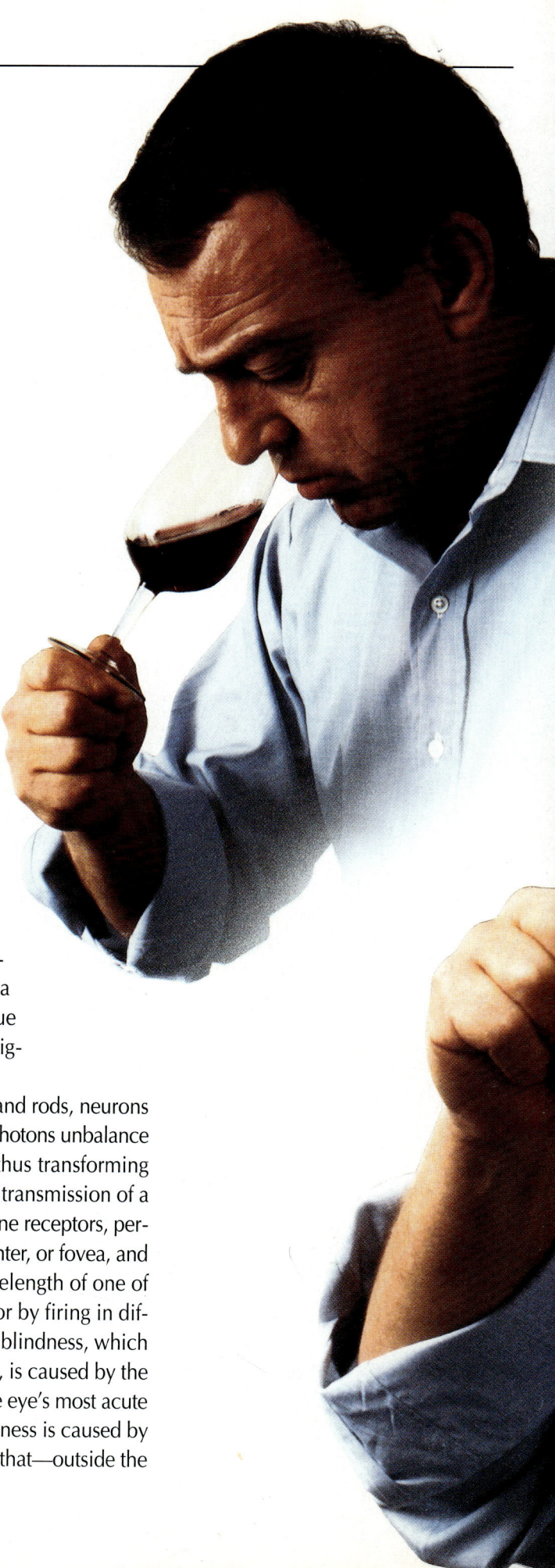

Human beings possess a brain that devotes more of itself to gathering and processing visual material than to any other sense. The starting point of sight is, of course, a pair of more-or-less round eyeballs. Each is about an inch in diameter, plumped with clear fluid, and coordinated in bony sockets by a collection of finely tuned muscles. But the true sensory story takes place behind the scenes.

Before light even reaches the retina, the convex curve of the cornea—the outermost window of the eyeball—refracts the entering light rays inward toward the center of the eye. Like a camera, the eye "sees" when light reflecting off an object passes through the transparent cornea and lens, which focus an inverted and reversed image of the object on the rear wall of the eyeball. But where the camera looks at the world through a single aperture, the eyes have the advantage of binocular sight that provides depth perception. And where the camera employs light-sensitive film, the eye uses a layer of nerve tissue called the retina, a branch office of the brain that carries out a significant amount of visual processing on its own.

When light rays reach the retina they are detected by cones and rods, neurons named for their distinctive shapes. Units of light intensity called photons unbalance the delicate electrochemical status quo of the receptor cells, thus transforming radiant energy into an electrochemical signal. The result is the transmission of a message to neuron bundles that exit the eye. The short, thick cone receptors, perhaps six million in all, are concentrated mostly in the retina's center, or fovea, and are responsible for color vision. Variously sensitive to the wavelength of one of three colors—blue, green or red—they code the shades of color by firing in different combinations of the three with varying frequency. (Color blindness, which affects 8 percent of the male population and almost no females, is caused by the absence or malfunction of certain cones.) Cones also provide the eye's most acute vision, and their total loss produces legal blindness. Night blindness is caused by the loss of the second type of photoreceptor, the long, thin rods that—outside the

STAYING ALIVE

GOOD TASTE

Winetasters who enjoy their work—and most do—avoid head colds. Without smell, even the most "muscular" wine is tired and flat. A true aficionado would dismiss it as having "no nose." Connoisseurs use more than 100 such terms, yet taste buds distinguish only four categories. Taste (red) and smell (blue) together are greater than the sum of their parts.

fovea—outnumber cones by ten to one. An estimated 125 million rods serve primarily in peripheral vision and in situations where light is of too low an intensity to excite the cones' firing system. Sometimes night vision is more acute if the eyes are trained on the side of an object, since the highest concentration of rods is just beside the cone-rich central retina. Because rods sense light in only black, white and shades of gray, it is often hard to distinguish color at night.

Nerve fibers converge in the optic nerve at the back of each eye. Less than half an inch from the point at which the left and right optic nerves set out on their mission from eye to brain, the two trunk lines meet at a crossing point called the optic chiasm. Here, in a shunting operation of amazing intricacy, half of the fibers from

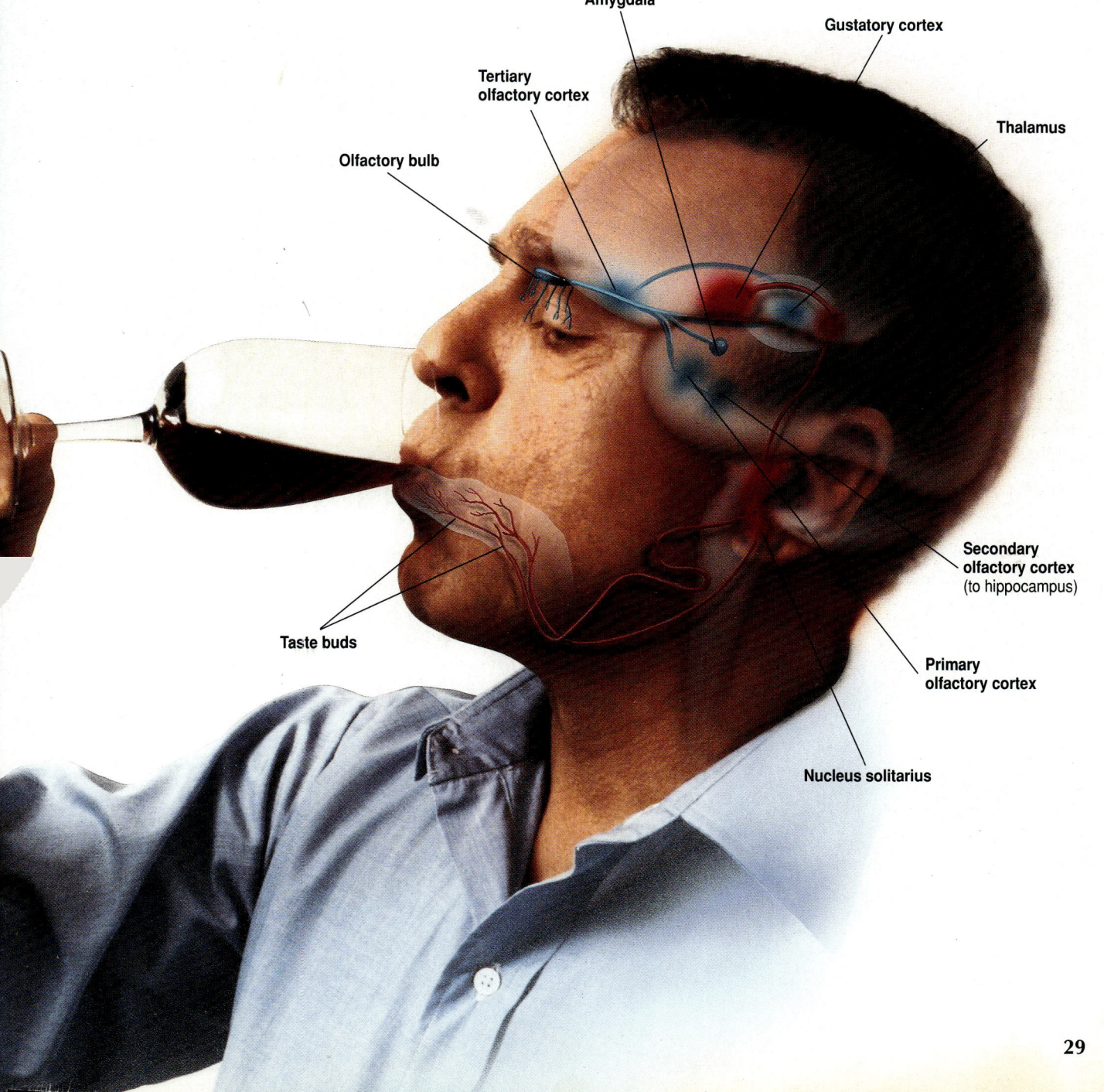

each optic nerve cross to join the remaining fibers of the opposite nerve. The rerouting is far from random. The fibers that cross are those linked to receptors closest to the nose. As a result, the visual messages that ultimately reach the visual cortex in each hemisphere are neatly divided. The left optic tract carries data to the left hemisphere from the right side of the field of vision. The right optic tract reports to the right hemisphere about the left visual field. En route to the visual cortex, axons of the optic tract pass through one of two processing structures. One, the superior colliculus, unites visual information with auditory and bodily information to coordinate head and eye movements in response to a stimulus.

The visual cortex is made up of millions of highly specialized "feature detector" cells, each one equipped to perceive a single visual quality such as shape, movement or orientation (vertical, horizontal or oblique). Tests show that kittens, exposed only to vertical lines during their early development, remain forever blind to other, nonvertical, lines. The cortex also compares "live" visual patterns to remembered patterns to help make sense of what is being seen. Cells in the visual cortex may hold a "trace" of an object that has been seen before. Experiments with monkeys reveal that single cells in this region respond to specific monkey faces recognized by the test monkey. And in yet another impressive process, the cortex completes binocular vision, forging two slightly different two-dimensional images into one three-dimensional, stereoscopic view, then analyzes the differences between them to arrive at a perception of the object's distance and size.

From an evolutionary point of view, the chemical senses—taste and smell—are among man's oldest and most primitive, but they pale in comparison to those of most animals. Taste relies for its initial impulse on chemical receptors. The specialized neurons are taste buds, bundles of about 50 cells each. These buds, totaling perhaps 5,000 throughout the mouth, cluster at the bases of the tiny red bumps, or papillae, on the surface of the tongue, and to a lesser extent on the palate, tonsils and throat. Each bud is sensitized to one of four primary tastes: sweet, salty, sour or bitter. And while all four kinds of buds are found all over the mouth, there is a tendency for each kind to concentrate in a particular sector of the tongue. Sweet sensors are located chiefly on the tip, sour on the sides, and bitter at the back of the tongue. But since few foods are composed of only one primary taste, each gustatory experience becomes a kind of census-taking problem for the brain. A head cold is a quick reminder of how weak the sense of taste is without aromatic cues. In fact, tests show that 50,000 times the usual amount of alcohol is required to identify its taste if the olfactory system is blocked.

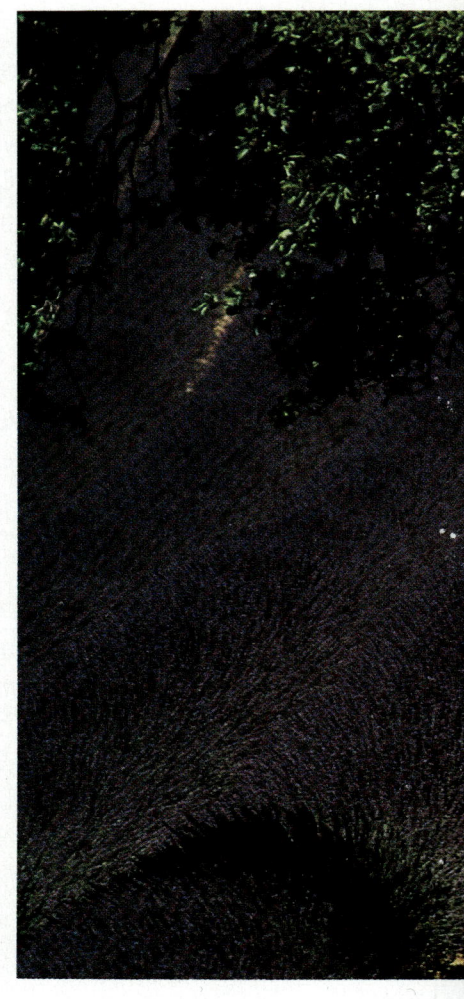

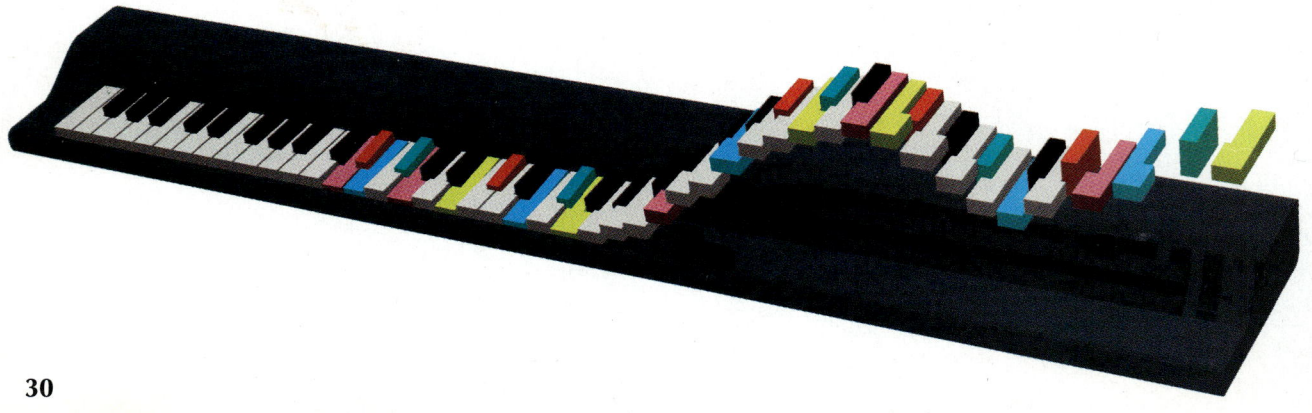

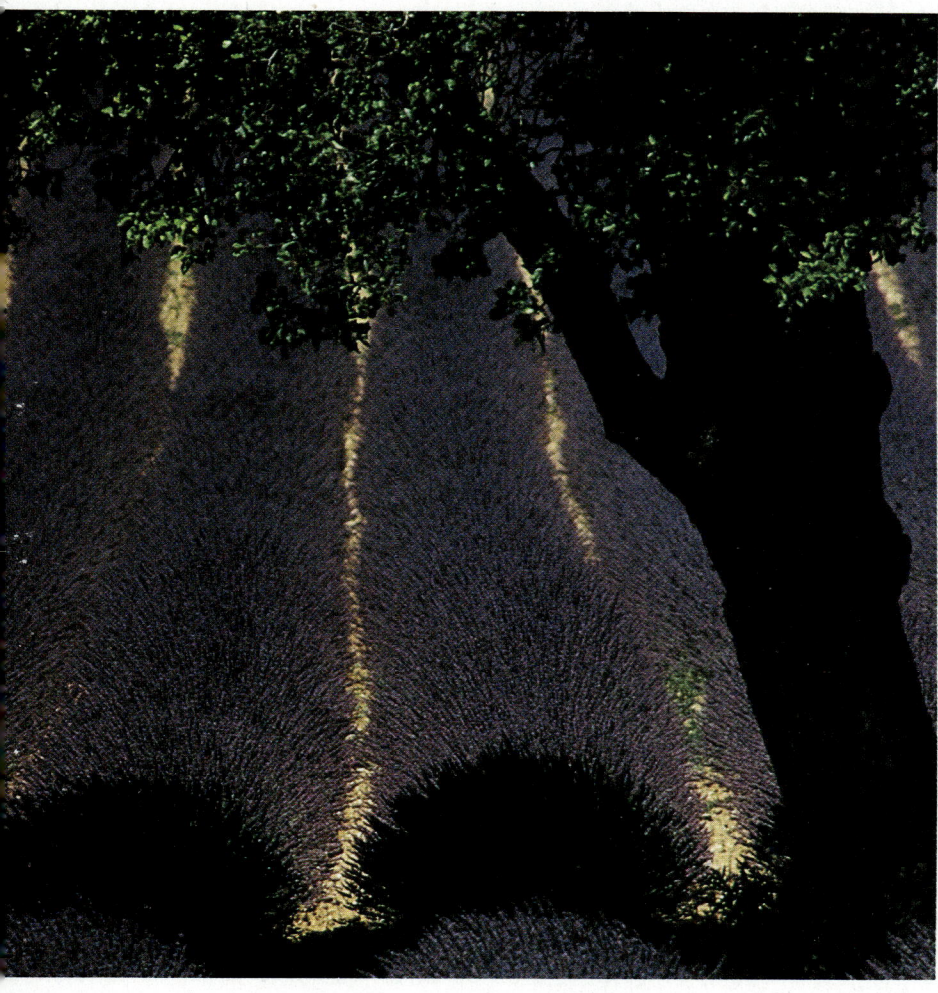

MAKING SCENTS

Even for an adult, the smell of baby powder can summon instant childhood feelings of comfort. A psychological triad is created from smell, emotion and memory because olfaction is physiologically linked to the limbic system, which is responsible for mood. Experiments indicate that many scents have biochemical properties that can stimulate or relax. Lavender and jasmine—even in subliminal doses—soothe, as do chamomile and peppermint. Rosemary and scarlet sage, which irritate the nose's trigeminal nerve, seem to stimulate by boosting production of adrenaline. Well-chosen aromas sprayed in factories and offices at the low-key level of elevator music may one day be employed to increase productivity or reduce stress.

The mood-altering aroma of lavender fields would certainly have an effect on the emotion-linked brain centers, even though humans have less scent sensibility than their mammalian ancestors.

SYNESTHESIA

Russian composer Rimsky-Korsakov suffered from synesthesia, a mingling of the senses. For him, the key of F major was green; A major was red. Other synesthetes insist that the taste of licorice sounds squeaky or that pronunciation of the letter M feels like damp moss. Some scientists believe that this condition—slightly more common among epileptics—represents a perceptual throwback that could shed light on the evolution of the senses.

The mechanism of taste depends on the translation of a chemical signal into an electrochemical one. Substances must first be soluble in water (or saliva), so that molecules can bind to the surface of a suitable receptor cell, producing an electrochemical change within. The coded electrochemical messages of taste travel to the brain by cranial nerves—channels of the peripheral nervous system leading to the brainstem. Along the way, some of the neurons communicate with the limbic system, giving rise to the theory that these roundabout pathways may play a role in linking memory and taste.

The sense of smell, or olfaction, originates in a pair of dime-sized, mucous-covered membranes tucked in cul-de-sacs just behind the bridge of the nose. Because the membranes are above and beyond the main pathway of air going to the lungs, ordinary breathing yields only a partial sensation of the environment's aromatic possibilities; it takes vigorous sniffing, which pulls more of the air into the chambers, to get the full measure of any olfactory experience.

Air is largely odorless nitrogen and oxygen, making the detection of smells tantamount to finding a needle in a haystack. The chemical particles of an odor vaporize and float through millions of air molecules. But a well-functioning human sense of smell can detect one molecule of pepper odor in a trillion molecules of air.

A dense mat of hairlike nerve endings rises up from the surface of more than 100 million receptor cells to capture odor molecules high in the nostrils. These nerve endings are unique for being the only parts of the brain that confront the external world directly. There an odorant-binding mucous collects vaporized molecules like flies on flypaper and receptor cells send electrochemical "smellograms" directly to a processing center. The first synapse in the pathway occurs in the olfactory bulb, deep in the forehead behind and above the eyes. From there the sensations travel to the cortex—only in smell is the cortex the first stop along the sensory pathway—then to several brain regions, including the amygdala, hypothalamus, thalamus, hippocampus and brainstem. Most of these areas are involved in the limbic system, accounting for the emotional and memory associations of smell. Smell, through the limbic system, also triggers remarkably strong libidinous and emotional reactions. Olfactory processing in the hypothalamus can set off visceral reactions such as nausea and hunger as well.

In much the same way as the visual system translates light into nerve impulses that inform sight, so the auditory system transforms waves of sound into the brain's electrochemical code. This masterpiece of engineering enables a healthy ear to detect a wide range of sound waves, oscillating between 20 cycles per second—below the lowest note on the piano—and 20,000 cycles per second—well above the highest note on a piccolo.

Sound waves, which travel in volleys of peaks and troughs, begin their journey to the brain through the external ear, then travel down an inch-long canal to strike the taut tympanic membrane, or eardrum, causing it to vibrate at the same rate as the arriving wave. Here the mechanical energy of the vibrating membrane sets in motion a tiny, delicate bone called the hammer. Then, in a pass-it-on sequence to two smaller bones and another membrane, the energy is amplified by about 50 times. On the other side of the last membrane, safely encased in some of the hardest and most protective bone in the body, is a unique, snail-shaped structure called the cochlea. This bony, fluid-filled organ constitutes the ear's transducer, turning the mechanical energy of the sound waves into the electrochemical codes understood by the brain.

The cochlea is equipped with thousands of hairlike sensory receptor cells. Fluid pressure waves, triggered by the incoming mechanical vibrations, stimulate the hair cells as they move through the spiral. The cells, which have no axons, communicate directly with neurons of the cochlear nerve. Energy is

CORTICAL NEIGHBORS
Neurons in the somatosensory band receive information originating outside the brain. The size of each segment relates directly to the amount of information being transmitted to the brain. Neurons in the adjacent motor cortex send messages destined for various body parts. Here segment size is related to the dexterity needed by that specific body part.

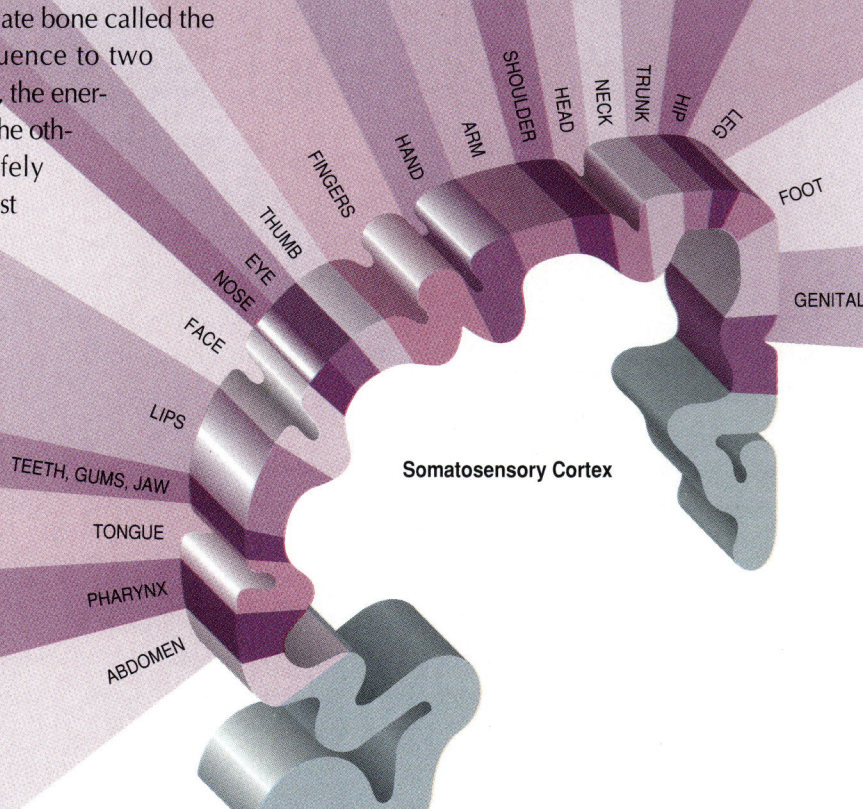

STAYING ALIVE

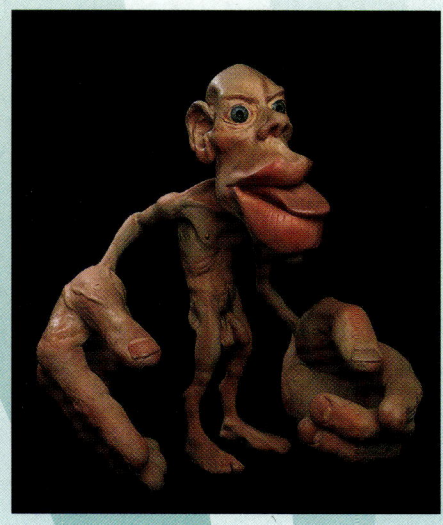

This sensory homunculus (little man) statue is a scale model showing bodily representation in the cortical band committed to the sense of touch. Lips and tongue, fingers and thumb rank high in tactile sensitivity.

translated once again, this time from mechanical to electrochemical form. The 30,000 relay neurons of the cochlear nerve make up a branch of the auditory nerve. From here, electrochemical signals undergo a long journey, with some neurons disembarking at subcortical stations, including the thalamus, and others traveling the entire route to the terminus—the primary auditory cortex, folded deep within major fissures in the right and left temporal lobes. The entire journey from start to finish has probably taken no more than one-fiftieth of a second.

The auditory brain relies on specific neurons to interpret qualities of sound such as pitch and loudness. Increments of volume are reflected in neurotransmitter release—the louder the noise, the greater the amount of transmitter released. The perception of certain types of sound—language, for example—is universal among humans. Even newborns are adept at distinguishing the human voice from other sounds, and the brain appears to be hard-wired to shunt speech to areas of the cortex dealing with language.

The inner ear is also the seat of sensory receptors for balance and the coordination of physical movement, eye movement and posture. Two distinct areas are responsible: the static labyrinth and the vestibular labyrinth. The static labyrinth consists of a pair of fluid-filled chambers located just above the cochlea. The static labyrinth monitors the body's position by means of flexible hair cells and minute ear stones—dense crystals whose motion bends the hair cell projections. This activity is translated into electrochemical messages that are sent via the acoustic cranial nerves to an area in the brainstem that signals various parts of the brain, including the cerebellum, the thalamus and the ocular nuclei. Information about the body's position allows eyes to keep a steady gaze while the body moves.

The vestibular labyrinth is made up of three semicircular canals that lie in three separate but perpendicular planes. They detect movement in three-dimensional space—side to side, up and down, backward and forward. When the data from all of the canals is combined, the brain gets a sense of the head's (and by implication, the body's) movement. This information, transferred along with data from the static labyrinth, is passed along to neurons in the cortex concerned with maintaining skeletal posture and movement. A major role of the cerebellum is to compare body position and movement with a constantly updated blueprint originating in neurons of the motor cortex. When weight is shifted from one foot to the other, commands are sent automatically from the brainstem, modulated by the cerebellum, to ensure balance.

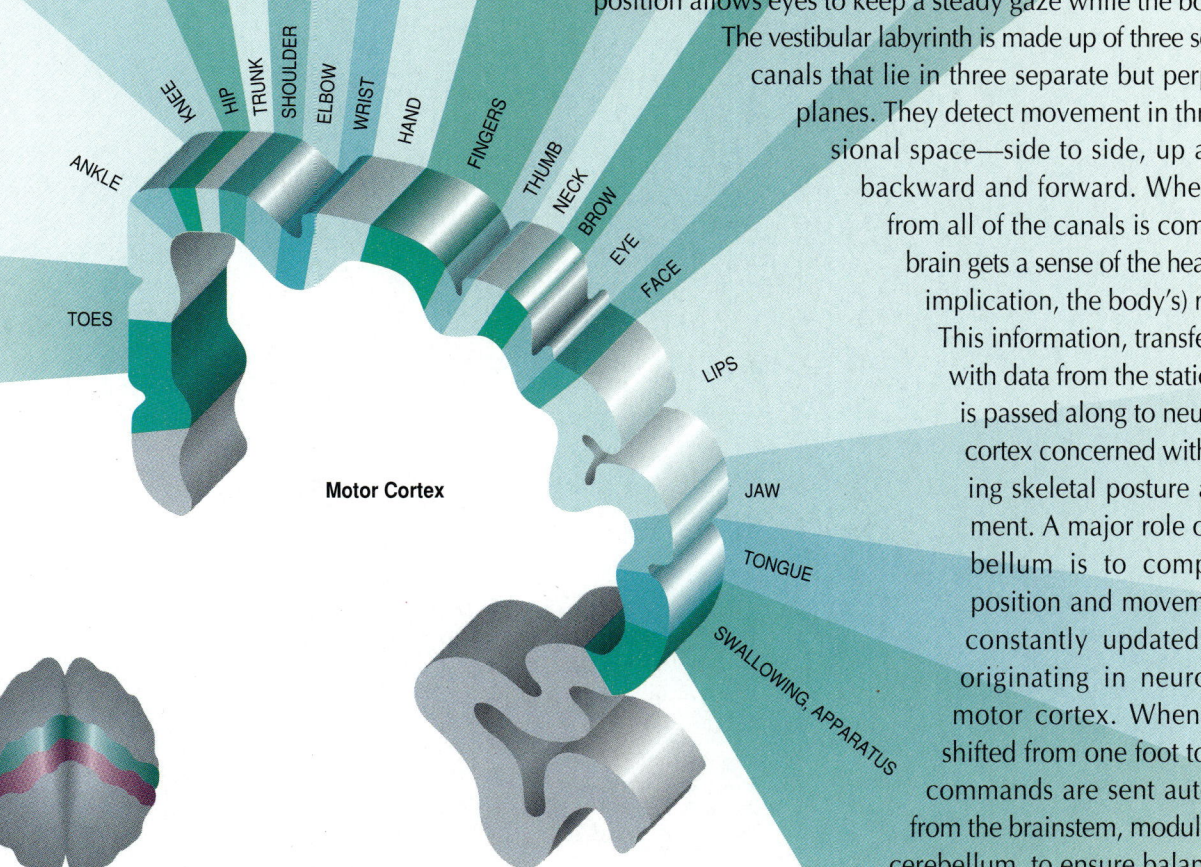

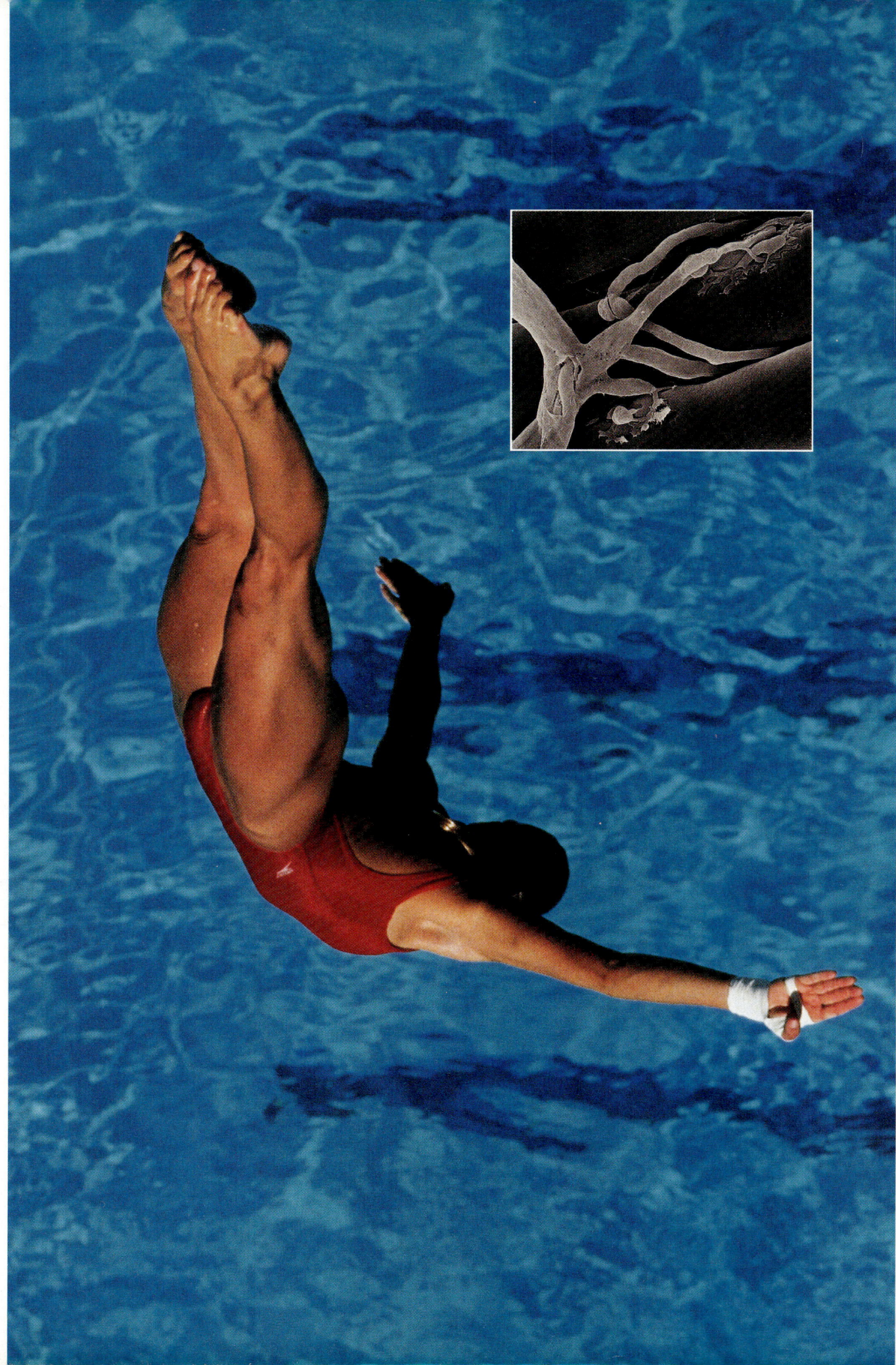

This perfectly executed dive owes its grace and power to complex neural mechanisms originating in the brain. Motor neurons, such as the one pictured here, relay instructions from the central nervous system to muscles.

Without the skin senses of touch, pain and temperature, the body would sustain injury and insult at virtually every turn. Skin receptors, though just as highly specialized as receptors in the other senses, are far more widely dispersed. The human skin—the largest organ of the body—measures 20 square feet on average and holds an estimated 640,000 receptors. Because the information provided by skin receptors is so varied, the receptor cells are distinguished by their variety and inventiveness. Each has its own cell structure and its own distribution pattern around the body, though many communication lines to the central nervous system are shared. When several different types lie close together, the mixed messages from them can be confusing. For example, a blow to the ulnar nerve at the elbow, commonly called the "funny bone," produces a mélange of painful, tingling, cold and warm sensations.

Among the skin receptors, the simplest in structure are the so-called free nerve endings—receptors for skin, muscle and joint pain. Some free nerve endings sense pricking or fast pain, transmitting pain signals at a moderate rate of 20 to 100 feet per second. Others recognize a slow or burning pain caused by deeper injury and transmit at a sluggish 1.5 to 6 feet per second. Either way, pain messages travel on an ascending pathway from the injury to the thalamus, where they are distinguished from other skin sensations and routed to the cortex for analysis. Associative neurons step in to add more information about the sensation, including how much pain the individual can tolerate based on past experiences.

The mechanism of peripheral pain sensation is thought to be related specifically to the stretching or distortion of nerve endings. When a needle punctures the skin, local tissue damage or distortion sets off a volley of electrochemical impulses. Chemical factors may amplify the pain sensations.

The skin, or somatic, senses are processed in an area of the brain's parietal lobe called the somatosensory ("body sense") cortex. Here are localized a sequence of distinct neural points corresponding to virtually every part of the body. As a result of research done by noted neurosurgeon Wilder G. Penfield at the Montreal Neurological Institute in the 1930s and 1940s, it was discovered that the pattern of distribution of these neural points is, in fact, an inverted map of the actual head-to-toe location of each body part. Penfield, noting this reverse correspondence, named this region the homunculus, or "little man." Terminals for pain and touch on the toes of the left foot are found at the very apex of the right sensory cortex; for the left calf and thigh a few inches farther along; for the hip, trunk, shoulder and arm, farther still. Almost the entire lower half of each sensory cortex is devoted to the eyes, nose, lips and tongue, a reflection of the relative density of the receptors in these areas and the amount of information they constantly transmit to the brain for processing.

GRACE IN SPACE

A mosquito hovering above the head of an intended victim is about to become a victim itself. Almost immediately, the brain initiates a learned strategy for self-defense. An arm is raised, palm extended, and at the moment the mosquito touches down, it is flattened.

Simple, perhaps. But the processing behind this voluntary motor response—calculating the speed and trajectory of the insect, the timing and the aim—is as wonderful as the sensory systems that provided the visual and auditory information about the mosquito's approach.

Indeed, motor and sensory functions—particularly tactile sensation—share elements of design. The primary cortical regions of movement and touch are neighbors: The motor cortex band lies in the frontal lobe, directly in front of the somatosensory band, which is in the parietal lobe. Neuron terminals in the two are distributed in a similar way, but with an interesting difference: The size of each section in the motor cortex corresponds not to the size of the body part served, but to the precision with which it must be controlled. Thus, the motor cortex—the thickest part of the cortex—gives a great deal of space to the neurons controlling the hands, lips and tongue, but relatively little to the neurons involved in moving parts of the shoulder or torso. And a good thing, too, for it is the dexterous facility of hands and mouth that gives humans their most distinctive skills: the ability to use tools and produce speech.

Voluntary movement occurs as a cooperative effort involving the motor cortex and many neural "consultants," including the premotor and supplementary motor

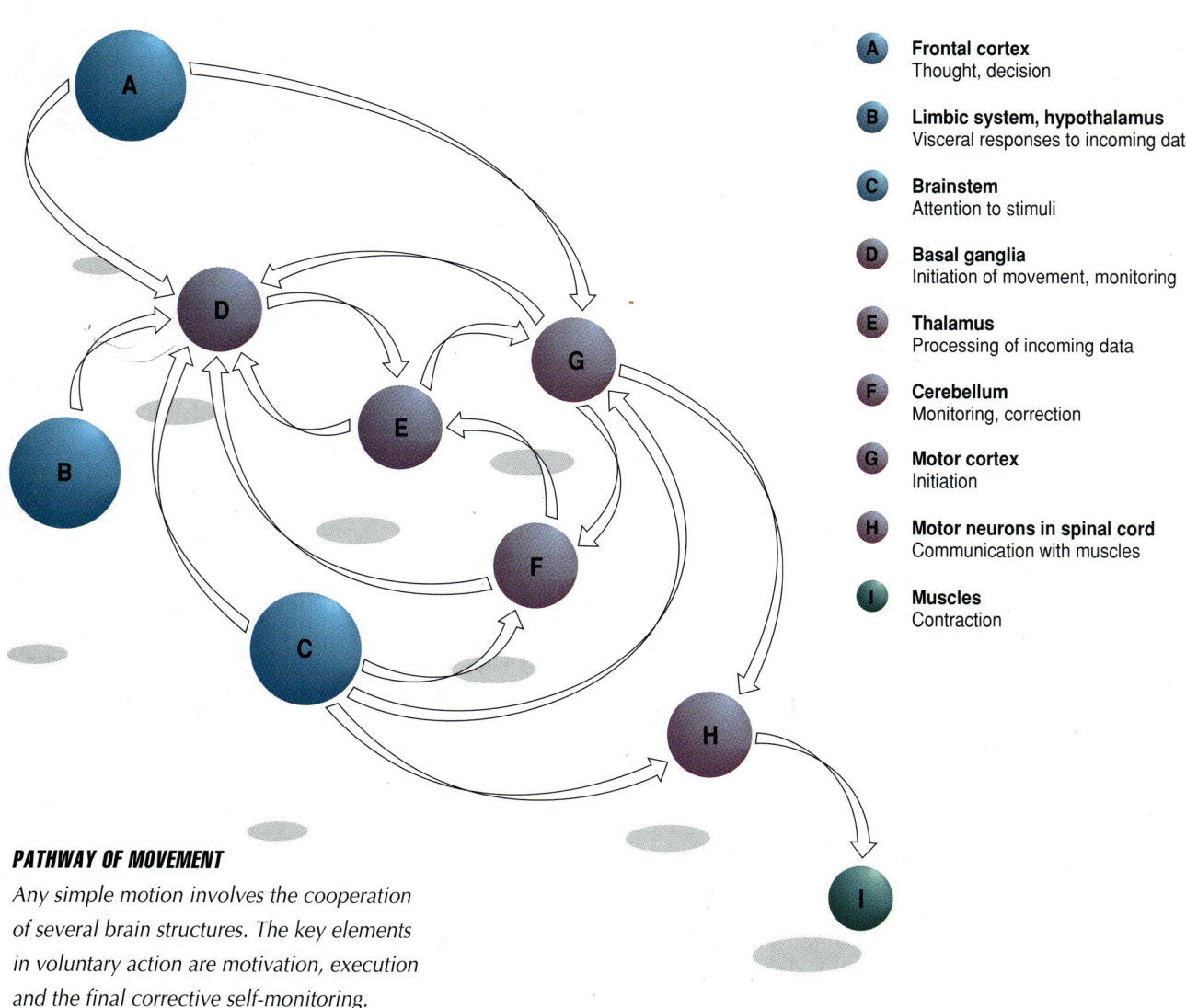

A Frontal cortex
Thought, decision

B Limbic system, hypothalamus
Visceral responses to incoming data

C Brainstem
Attention to stimuli

D Basal ganglia
Initiation of movement, monitoring

E Thalamus
Processing of incoming data

F Cerebellum
Monitoring, correction

G Motor cortex
Initiation

H Motor neurons in spinal cord
Communication with muscles

I Muscles
Contraction

PATHWAY OF MOVEMENT
Any simple motion involves the cooperation of several brain structures. The key elements in voluntary action are motivation, execution and the final corrective self-monitoring.

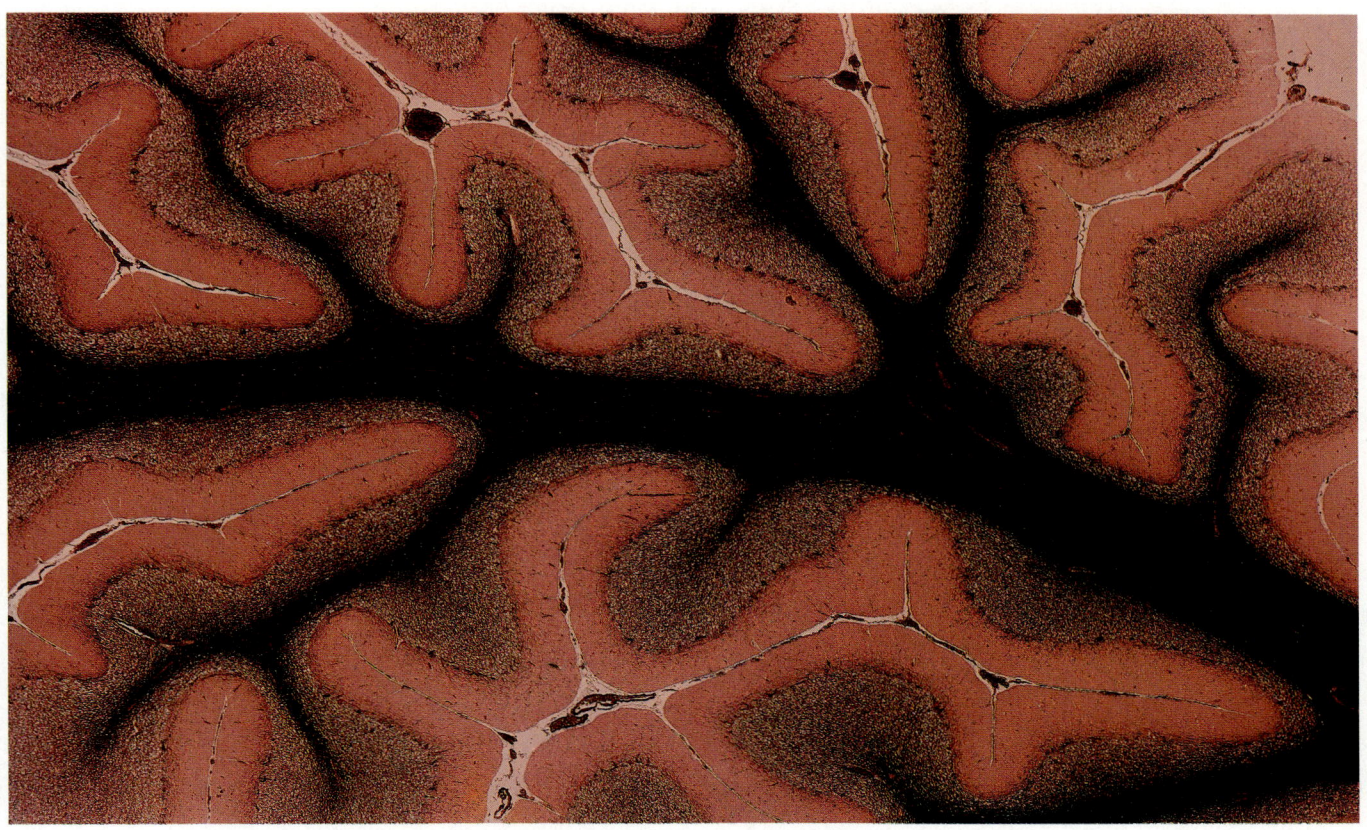

The cerebellum—showing its internal structure in this cross section—plays a crucial role in both the execution and refinement of movement. Feedback systems enable this "little brain" to compare ongoing actions with their motor cortex blueprint, correct the movement and then modify the brain's program for similar future actions.

area, the basal ganglia, and the cerebellum. The premotor cortex, located in the frontal lobe of the brain, is thought to be involved in the regulation of posture; it directs the motor cortex on the best body position for a specific body movement. The supplementary motor area, another tiny region in the frontal lobe, appears to influence the planning and initiation of movement based upon past experience. In fact, with the use of electroencephalographs (EEGs), which record brain activity, scientists can now see that the mere anticipation of a motion provokes neural firing in the supplementary region. The basal ganglia, nuclei found low in the forebrain, send back messages to the primary, supplementary and premotor areas of the cortex in order to coordinate gross motor movements—moving one leg in front of the other, for example—in a smooth and orderly fashion.

Complementing the basal ganglia, the cerebellum is in charge of fine-tuned movement—the kind that allows a surgeon to perform intricate repairs to a ruptured cornea or a diver to execute a full gainer with a double twist. This structure, sometimes called the "second brain," coordinates the start, execution and end of a physical act, helps to maintain balance and body tone, and is crucial in performing rapid and consecutive movements, such as playing the piano.

The cerebellum tracks the position of head and neck, trunk, arms and legs on the basis of raw data from "position-sense" receptors scattered throughout the body. Proprioception—the "sixth sense"—informs the individual of limb position and muscle tension, relying on information from hundreds of thousands of stretch receptors buried in muscles and tendons. Sensitive to movement, the receptors report to the brain about the position of limbs and body. The cerebellum uses the data to advise the motor cortex on its next move.

Motor Misfires

A little shakiness, trouble rising from a sitting position: The early stage of Parkinson's disease resembles normal aging. In time, balance is impaired, increased tremor interferes with eating or reading, and, most distressing, the body refuses to do the mind's bidding. Advanced parkinsonism is signaled by episodes of "freezing" in mid-movement, deadpan face, emotionless voice and a characteristic tremor that worsens when the muscles are inactive.

Every voluntary bodily action results from a multitude of electrochemical signals in the brain. At no time is this more evident than when the crucial chemical balance is upset. Too much or too little of a neurotransmitter such as dopamine can cause severe impairment. This is the case in parkinsonism and Huntington's chorea.

A conglomeration of neurons in the basal ganglia, called the substantia nigra, links the brain's thought centers and the muscles themselves. Responsible, in part, for initiating movement, the pigmented cells of the substantia nigra (black substance) use dopamine to dispatch orders from the cerebral cortex. In parkinsonism, key dopamine-producing neurons mysteriously die, leaving behind characteristic markers known as Lewy bodies and cutting lines of communication. Fortunately a drug called L-dopa, which replenishes dopamine in the basal ganglia, reduces immobility and tremor.

Unfortunately, excessive doses of L-dopa can produce symptoms similar to those of Huntington's chorea, an ultimately fatal disorder resulting from too much dopamine. Cell death in a structure called the caudate nucleus, also part of the basal ganglia, results in a drunken gait, involuntary dance-like movements, drooling and slurred speech. In early stages, Huntington's patients are sometimes accused of intoxication. As the disease progresses, characteristic jerking and writhing movements become more prominent.

Huntington's is not yet treatable by medication, though a genetic marker has been identified, enabling early detection and creating hopes that in the future genetic manipulation may save carriers of the faulty gene. An exciting area of Parkinson's research involves grafting healthy dopamine-producing cells into the unhealthy brain.

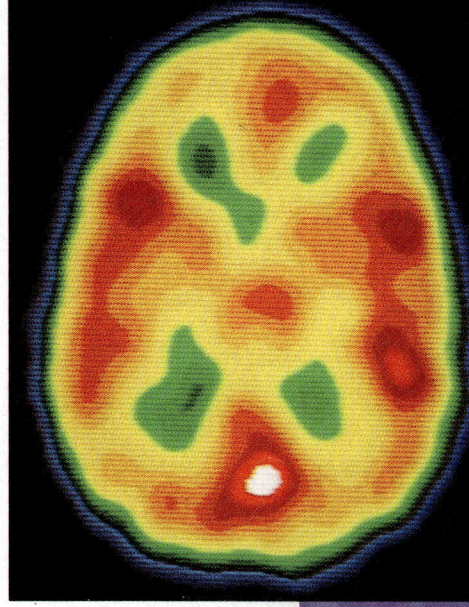

PET scans contrast the crippling effect of neural death in Parkinson's disease (below) *with the balanced image of the healthy brain* (right). *Microphotography captures the telltale Parkinson's signature—Lewy bodies occupying the neuron* (opposite).

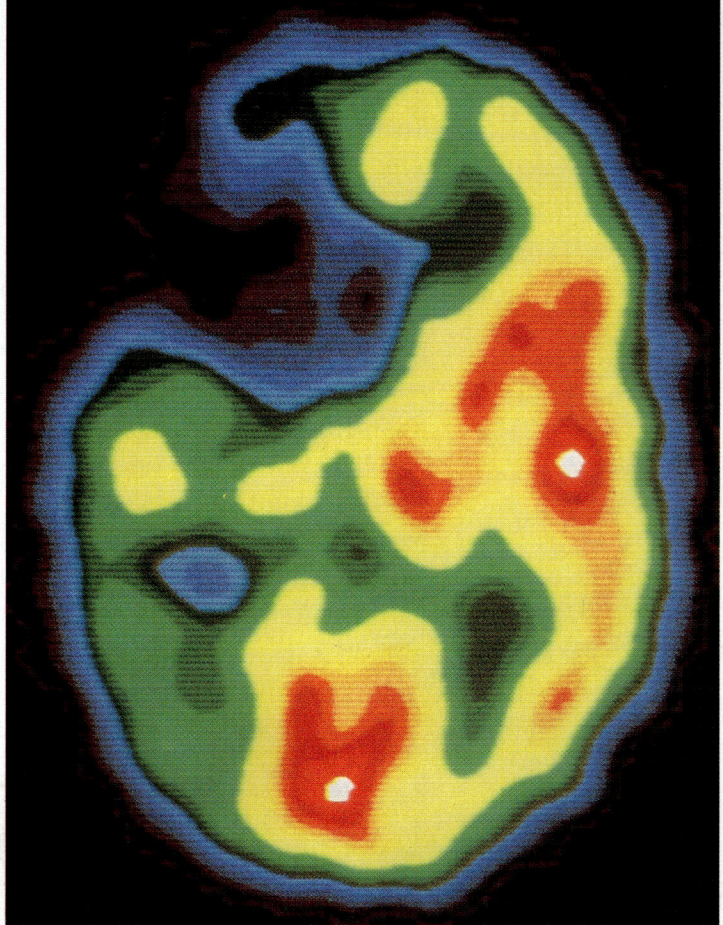

STAYING ALIVE

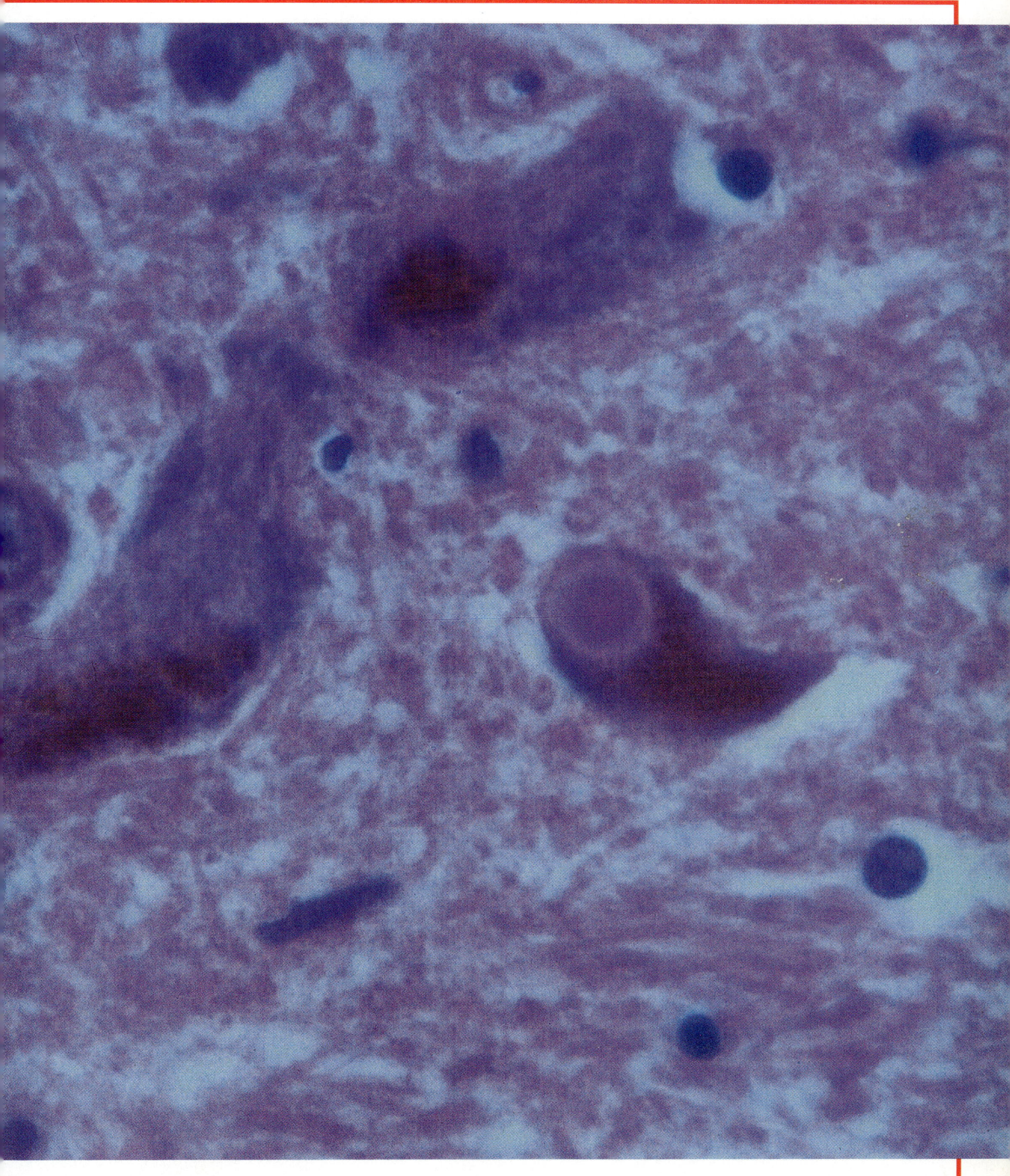

Once a program of action is initiated, the motor cortex sends impulses along descending, or efferent, neural fibers into the medulla oblongata. Most cross to the opposite side of the CNS, and travel downward until they communicate with a second, "lower," motor cell nucleus. This may be in the brainstem (if the impulses are involved in moving parts of the face and head), or in the spinal cord (if the motor unit involved moves neck, shoulders, torso or limbs). Here the motor neuron's axon makes a beeline for a group of muscle fibers within a specific muscle. Just short of its destination, the nerve fiber branches out, forming junctions with numbers of muscle fibers. Electrochemical messages arriving at these locations cause release of the neurotransmitter acetylcholine. This chemical spurs the muscle fibers to contract, thus initiating movement. The instructions are simply "on" or, by default, "off." Most of the 650-odd muscles in the body are paired in opposition—one for extending, the other for flexing. (In a condition called dystonia, interfering signals command extension and flexing at the same time, resulting in a series of contortions.) And each of these muscles is wired in such a way that groups of muscle fibers can be operated in seemingly infinite combinations to produce fine motor control. Research shows that physical skills are refined and stored not in the physical machinery of muscles, tendons and bones, but in the brain—particularly the cerebellum. Remarkably, mental rehearsal of sport or musical skills has proved almost as effective as physical practice. Such an integral role is played by the brain in any physical activity that the visualization of a ski jump, for example, elicits EEG-measurable electrochemical activity in muscles. Since its discovery, visuomotor behavior rehearsal (or VMBR) has become a common practice among Olympic athletes.

SURVIVAL OF THE SPECIES

Anatomists generally do not speak of the brain as a reproductive organ, but from an evolutionary point of view, almost no other function is more important than the brain's role in controlling sexual behavior. Without this, the human species would not survive from one generation to the next. The primary control center of most sexually related activities is the hypothalamus. However, it is via the pituitary gland that the hypothalamus directs hormones governing reproduction, sexual development and behavior.

Though the sex of every fetus is determined genetically at the moment of conception, sexual anatomy begins to develop between the sixth and eighth week of gestation. During this period, male genes initiate the formation of testes from the embryonic gonads. The testes soon begin to secrete hormones, called androgens, that masculinize the reproductive tract. In the female, the embryonic gonads become ovaries, and in the absence of testicular hormones, external female genitals develop. As well as affecting male sexual organs, testicular hormones also guide development of the brain, leading to gender-related differences in the hypothalamus and other brain structures. In addition, exposure to the androgen testosterone in prenatal and early postnatal life appears to change the way the nervous system responds to hormones after puberty.

There is increasing evidence that sex-linked hormones play a role in shaping some behavioral and cognitive differences between males and females. Although it is hard to determine which behaviors are hormone-related and which are

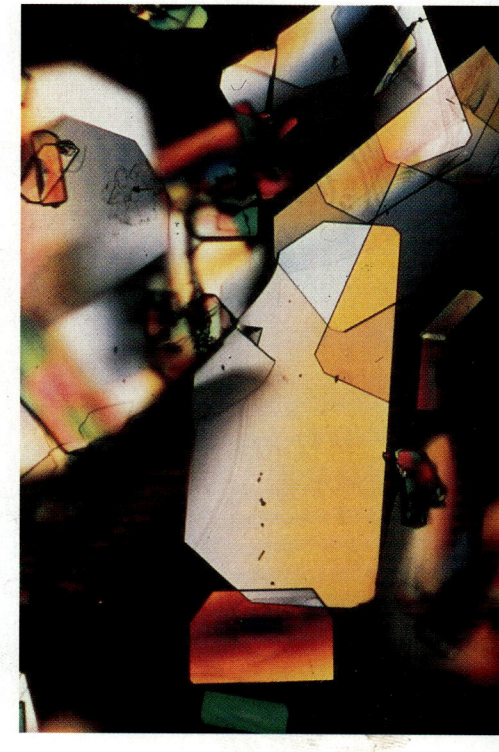

Hormones—here in crystal form—affect not only sexual development, but also the formation of the fetal brain. While so-called "male" and "female" hormones occur in both genders, greater concentrations of progesterone (below) and estrogen (bottom) are found in females, while testosterone (right) predominates in males.

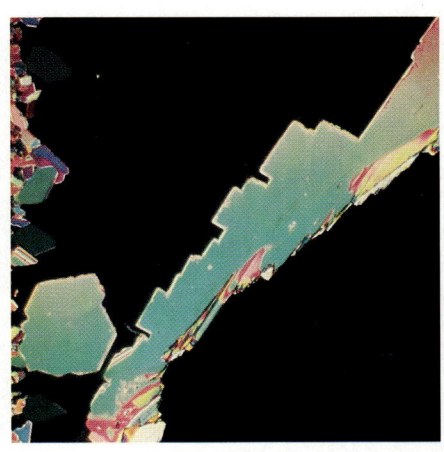

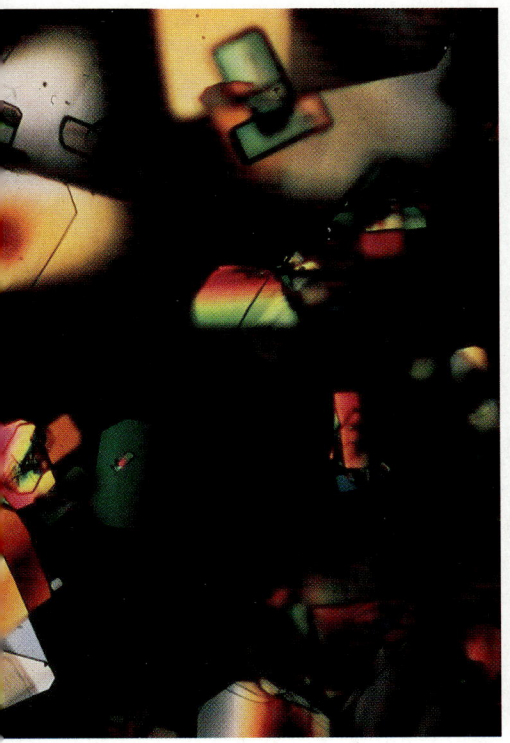

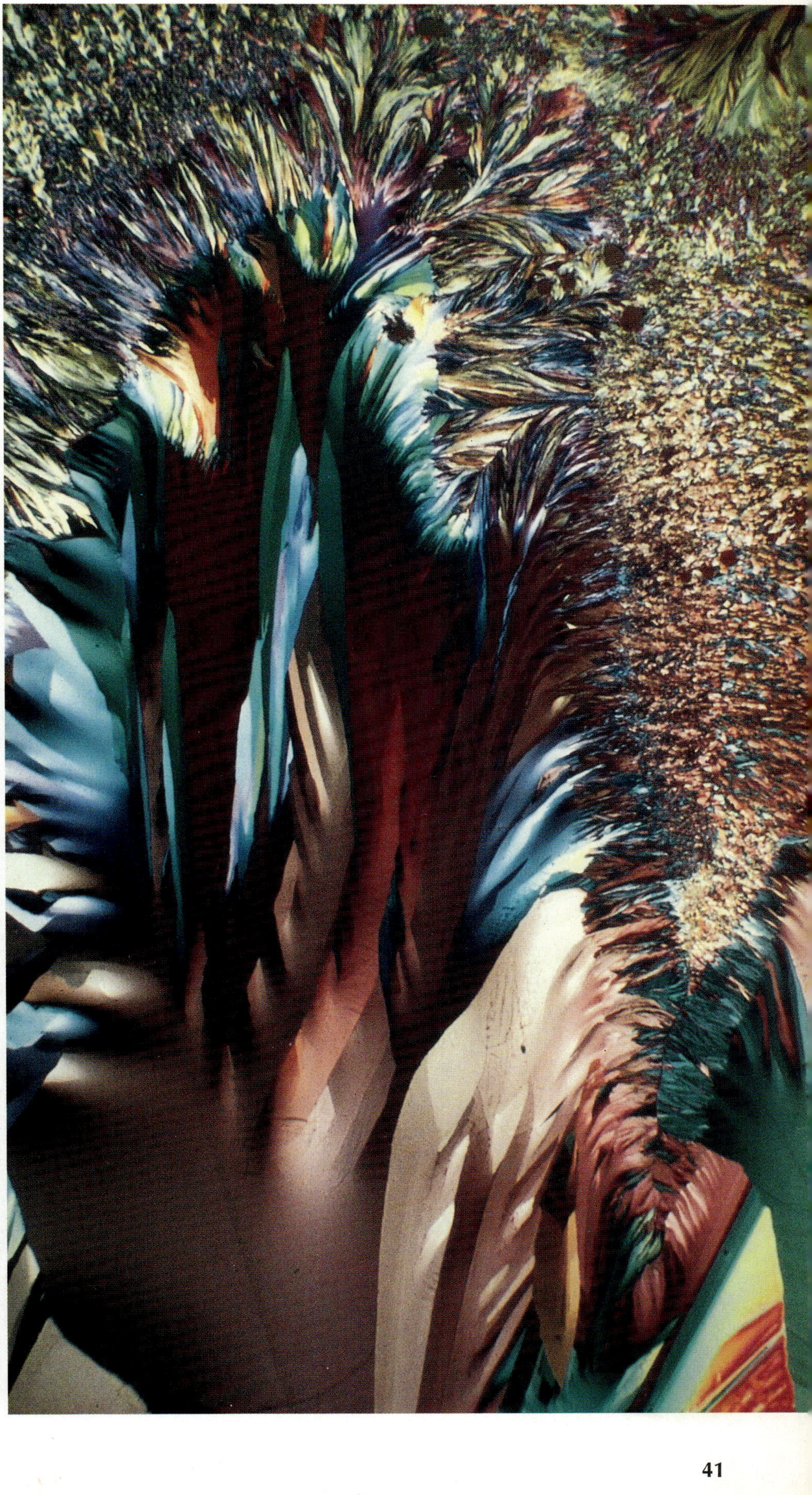

learned, hormone exposure before birth might affect how males and females respond to their environment after birth. Some studies suggest that right from infancy girls are more responsive to social contexts than to other kinds of stimuli. Girls tend to demonstrate more "parenting rehearsal" behavior, the kinds of activities associated with doll play. On the other hand, boys respond as much to "things" as to human stimulation, a pattern quite different from that of girls. Boys also tend to be more active and physically aggressive than girls throughout childhood, and to have greater gross motor control.

Sexual dimorphism is, of course, just the opening phase of the brain's contribution to sexuality. Through the hypothalamus the brain coordinates the biochemistry of sexual maturation in puberty; manages many of the psychosocial patterns of human mating behavior; controls the timetable of female ovulation, conception and pregnancy; and plays several roles in keeping men and women sexually active throughout their lives.

Once again, it is hormones and the brain's autonomic system that make the body do the brain's bidding. The process begins when neurons in the hypothalamus produce the gonadotropin-releasing hormone (GnRH) that is released into the blood and carried directly to the pituitary gland. There it causes the release of luteinizing hormone (LH) and follicle-stimulating hormone (FSH), which are in turn carried in the bloodstream to the testes in males, the ovaries in females. Having arrived at these organs, the hormones stimulate reactions as different as the two sexes involved. In the testes, the LH sets off the production of testosterone, the predominant chemical factor in maintaining a wide range of masculine behaviors and secondary sex characteristics. FSH in the testes stimulates sperm production. In the ovaries, LH and FSH are essential in the production of the hormones estrogen and progesterone and in the cycle of ovulation and menstruation. These last hormones are directly responsible for maintaining female sex characteristics and such specialized functions as pregnancy, labor and delivery. Oxytocin activates the contraction of the uterus during the final stages of labor. Prolactin, a hormone produced by the pituitary, directs lactation and other maternal behaviors such as the instinctual desire to suckle the young. ("The pill," the most commonly used form of oral contraception, consists of a combination of estrogen and progesterone, whose levels in the bloodstream are kept constant in order to suppress the normal midcycle hormone surge that results in ovulation.)

Normal production of male or female hormones is a matter of ebb and flow. The hypothalamus, which is constantly monitoring the pituitary's work, directs the production of LH and FSH so that appropriate levels for daily and monthly cycles are produced. This ensures that sexuality remains at a fairly high pitch most of the time (as distinct from most other animals, in which sexual arousal, mating and conception are seasonal). But in case this is not enough to keep humans reproducing, other parts of the brain control accessory systems to fan the flames.

Sexual excitement results in the release of endorphins, the brain's natural opiates. The neural activity of sex produces, as a byproduct, intense but short-lived ecstasy. The autonomic nervous system makes an entry on the scene, too, causing speedups in blood flow, pulse, and heartbeat, as well as the spasmic muscle contractions of orgasm. And the senses contribute, the olfactory sense responding pleasurably to chemical sexual stimuli, including those contained in human sweat,

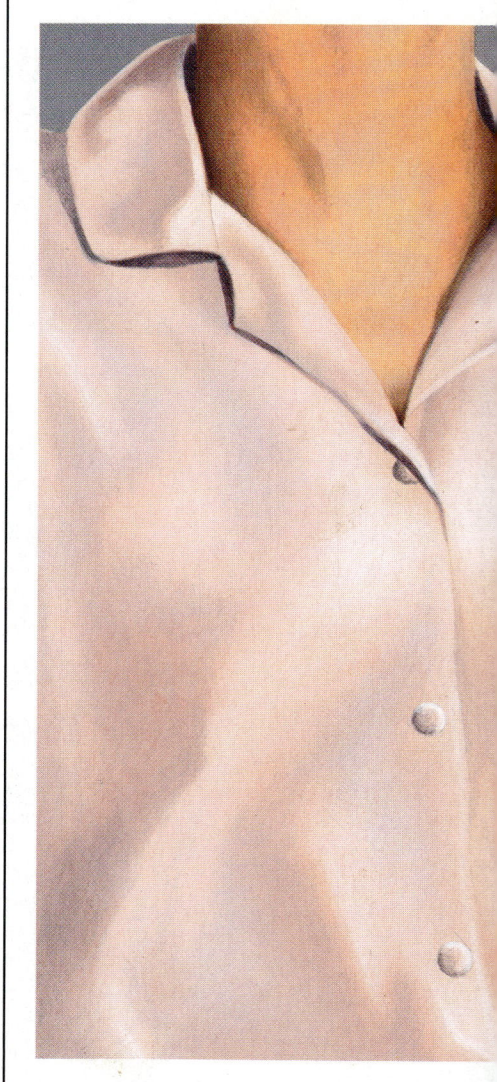

while the tactile receptors clustered around the genitals, breasts, mouth and lips respond positively to touch. But, favorable as these reactions are, they are all found to greater or lesser degree throughout the animal kingdom. It is in the realm of psychological arousal that humans are unique.

Desire appears to be in the eye (and brain) of the beholder when it comes to sexual matters. Erotic fantasies are sometimes enough to trigger the full panoply of autonomic responses that culminate in orgasm. By the same token, the physiological mechanisms underlying human sexual drive and potency can also be the victim of subversive psychological factors, including feelings of inadequacy, depression, inhibition and anxiety. Aphrodisiacs, not one of which has ever been proved to have intrinsic value in stimulating flagging desire, may work on the psychology of the believer. Perhaps because the user is able to put his faith in the aphrodisiac's power, he is able to override his own negative state of mind, freeing instinctive drives to take over.

The brain, it seems, overlooks very little in its continuing quest to keep the body—and the species—alive and well.

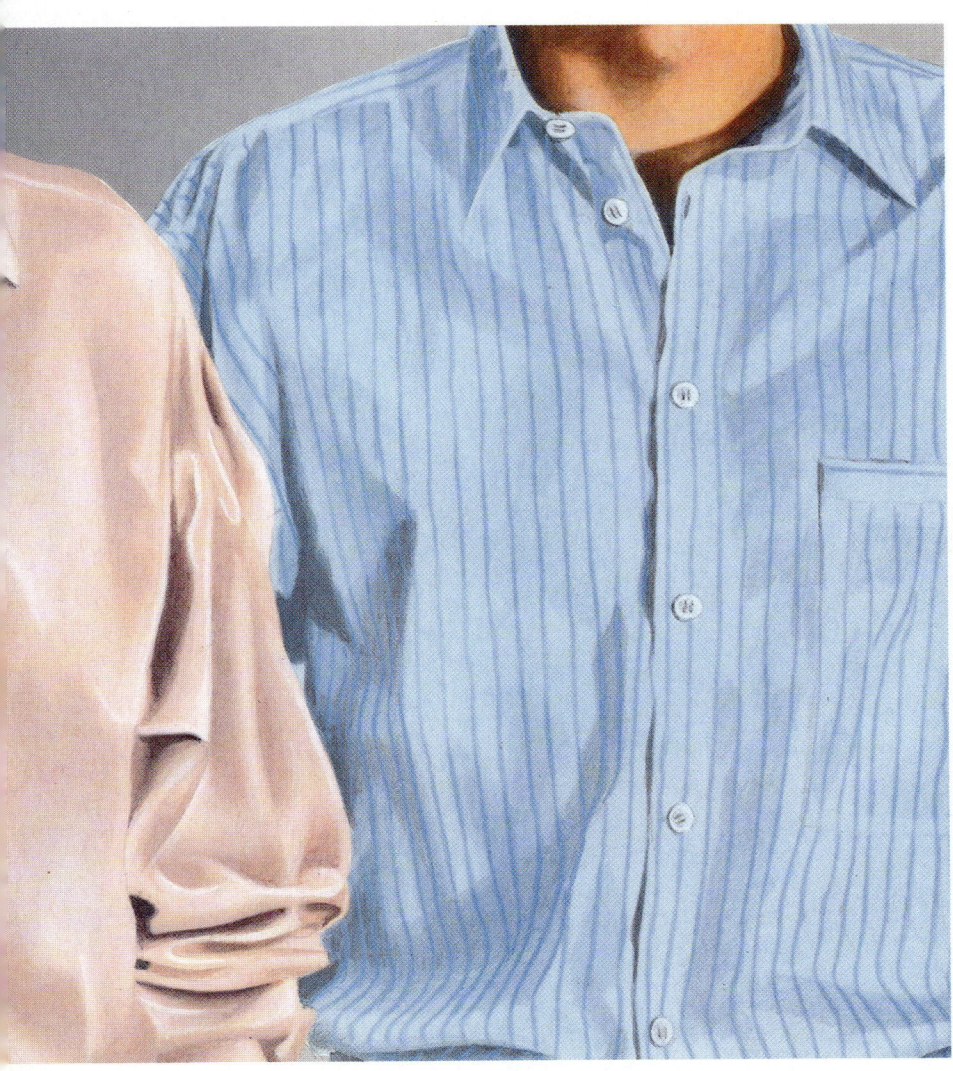

SEX ON THE BRAIN

No one knows to what extent sex roles are learned and to what extent they are innate, but scientists agree that males and females behave in clearly distinct ways. Males in all cultures are more aggressive than females, and at an early age. Females are earliest to develop finesse in language, logical thinking and fine motor coordination, while males excel in math and are better oriented in three-dimensional space. Even today, children are unconsciously schooled according to traditional roles, explaining part of the difference. Hormones might explain the rest.

Some researchers speculate that the androgen testosterone slows the development of the left hemisphere in males, while favoring the right hemisphere. Since language is a left-hemisphere function, this might explain girls' precociousness in speaking and women's generally higher scores on tests of verbal fluency. Right hemisphere dominance might explain the greater incidence of left-handedness in males (since motor signals cross to the opposite side of the body).

Intriguing male-female differences—some as minor as how clothes are buttoned—puzzle researchers. Some arise from learned behavior; others may have physiological roots.

The Detectives

Technology plays a huge role in the investigations of science and medicine into the workings of the brain. Aside from the need for tools that can uncover clues to the brain's hidden mysteries, there is the more practical and humane consideration of helping people with problems. The great strides taken in the last decade in both understanding function and improving diagnosis and treatment have come about through this productive partnership of inquiring science and ingenious technology. Three of the most impressive advances involve taking scans of the brain. They provide neuroscientists with an inside view of this complex structure at work.

MRI

An accident victim stares up at the seamless metal cocoon, oblivious to the chemical square dance being performed in her brain. In what seems to be X-ray vision without X-rays, a magnetic resonance imaging (MRI) scanner exposes her brain to a harmless magnetic field. Hydrogen-rich water is the main ingredient in nerve cells and the magnetic field of the scanner causes the positively charged protons of hydrogen molecules to tilt like tiny magnets. Then, as the magnetic field is shut off, a television monitor displays radio wave resonance emitted as the protons re-orient themselves. The resulting image displays brain matter and even distinguishes between different types of tissue. The accident victim can rest easy; the readout shows that her brain is unharmed.

Magnetic resonance imaging picks up where CT (CAT-scan) technology left off, slicing the living brain at a variety of depths and angles, and cutting through the visual "noise" created by CT's sensitivity to bone. Brain tumors, blocked by the skull in CT scans, are readily visible through MRI. Although CT retains some advantages, MRI's striking contrast of gray and white matter enables clinicians to zero in on virtually any region desired, making it the diagnostic tool of choice in most brain disease.

Certain AIDS-related disorders are now being spotted without penetrating the skull,

---

A patient enters the smooth walls of an MRI tunnel. The scanning process takes just minutes, causes no discomfort and has no reported harmful effects. Doctors and scientists are provided with stunningly clear images of brain tissue such as the one below of a healthy brain.

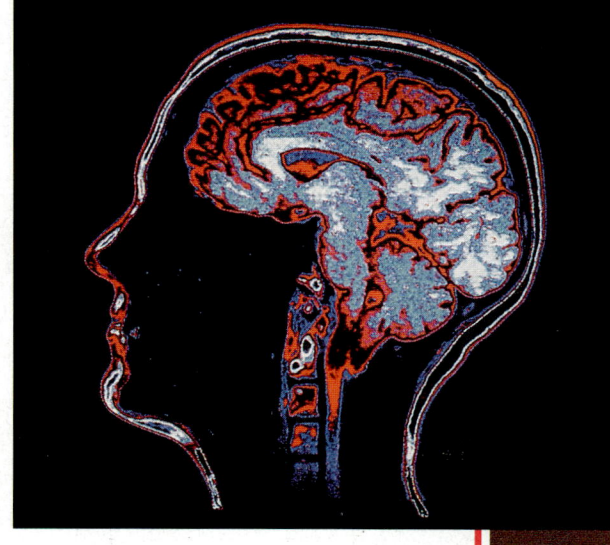

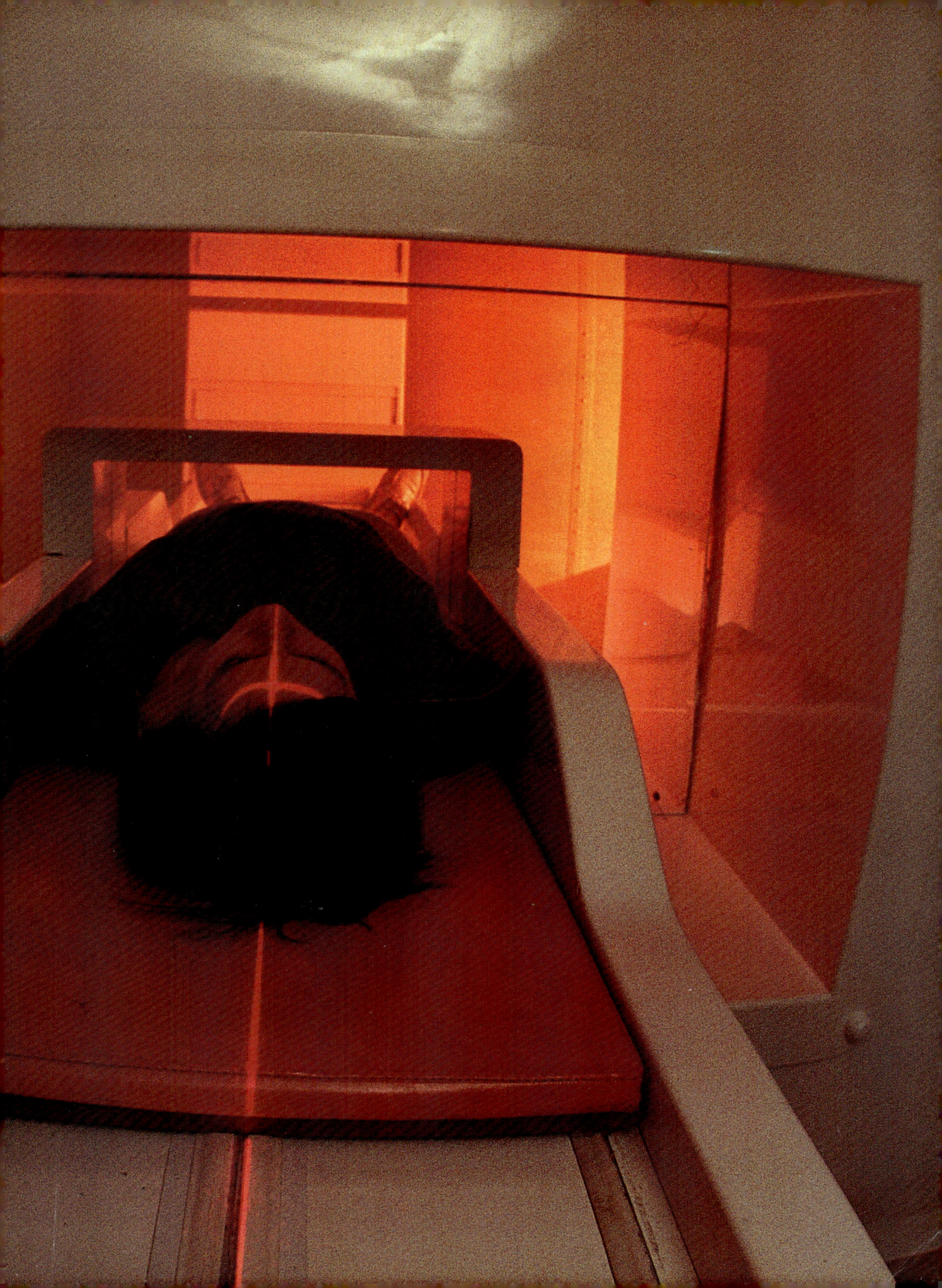

as are the tiny hemorrhages caused by concussions. Swelling or cell death, associated with tumors, strokes and multiple sclerosis, also are MRI-identifiable because of their unusual water content.

The superb anatomical map generated by MRI is often used in conjunction with other kinds of brain imaging. The chemical or electrical activity registered by other scanners is easier to localize when oriented by an MRI image.

PET

Symptoms ranging from seizures to aural hallucinations have brought a nervous and muddled patient to the mechanized bench in front of a positron emission tomography (PET) scanner. In lucid moments the patient has recalled a number of disturbing incidents over recent months—suddenly forgetting a familiar telephone number, losing track in mid-conversation—occurrences that in retrospect seem related to the hallucinations and seizures. Now the bench begins to move slowly forward until the patient's head lies within the hole of the large doughnut-shaped scanner.

Nearby, the problem reveals itself on the screen of a monitor, in dynamic color. A map of the man's brain shows a quivering topography of red islands, bordered by concentric rings of orange, yellow and green in a sea of blue. Then, off to one side, a white spot surrounded by lifeless black. The neuroscientist studying the image knows that white indicates bad news for this patient—ravenous consumption of glucose, gluttonous behavior required to feed the rampant cell growth of a brain tumor.

PET has emerged as one of the most promising applications of nuclear medicine. Unlike MRI, whose valuable contribution is a reliable picture of tissue, PET gives a live show, a moving picture of biochemical activity within the brain.

The process relies on the fact that radioactive substances called isotopes lose half their radioactivity within minutes or hours. The dissipating radioactivity results in the release of positrons. Each positron collides with an electron, and the two particles annihilate each other, releasing a pair of gamma rays. A PET scanner detects the gamma rays, calculates their source and locates it on a monitor.

To study the brain's consumption of a substance such as glucose, a small amount of radioisotope is used as a tag and injected into the bloodstream. The marked substance

This PET scan of a healthy brain (above) shows a symmetrical balance of metabolic activity. Hot colors indicate biochemical communication, while cool hues represent neuronal quiet. Researchers use these color maps to localize functions to specific regions.

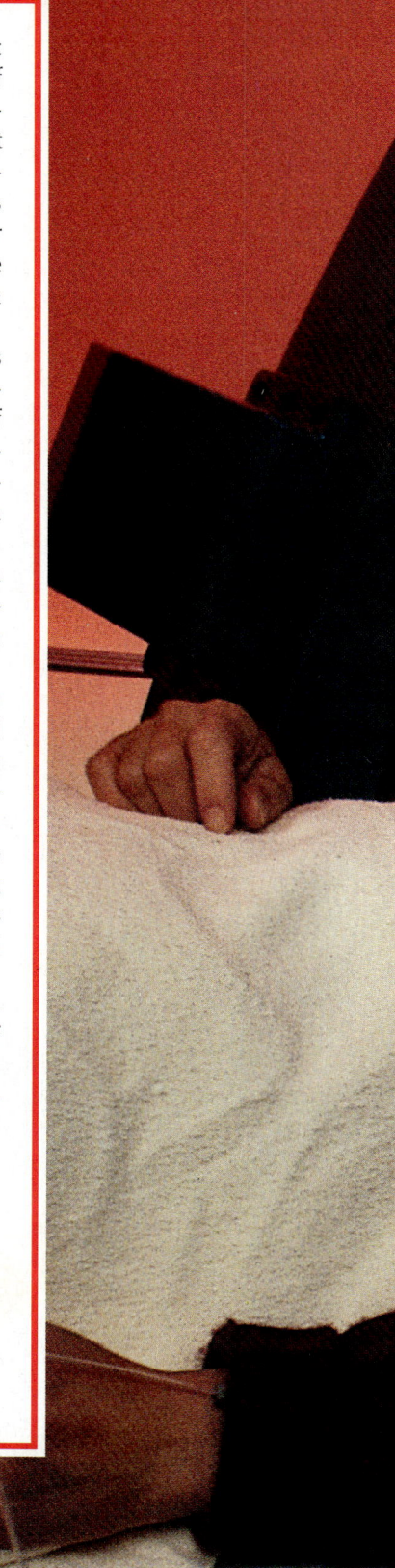

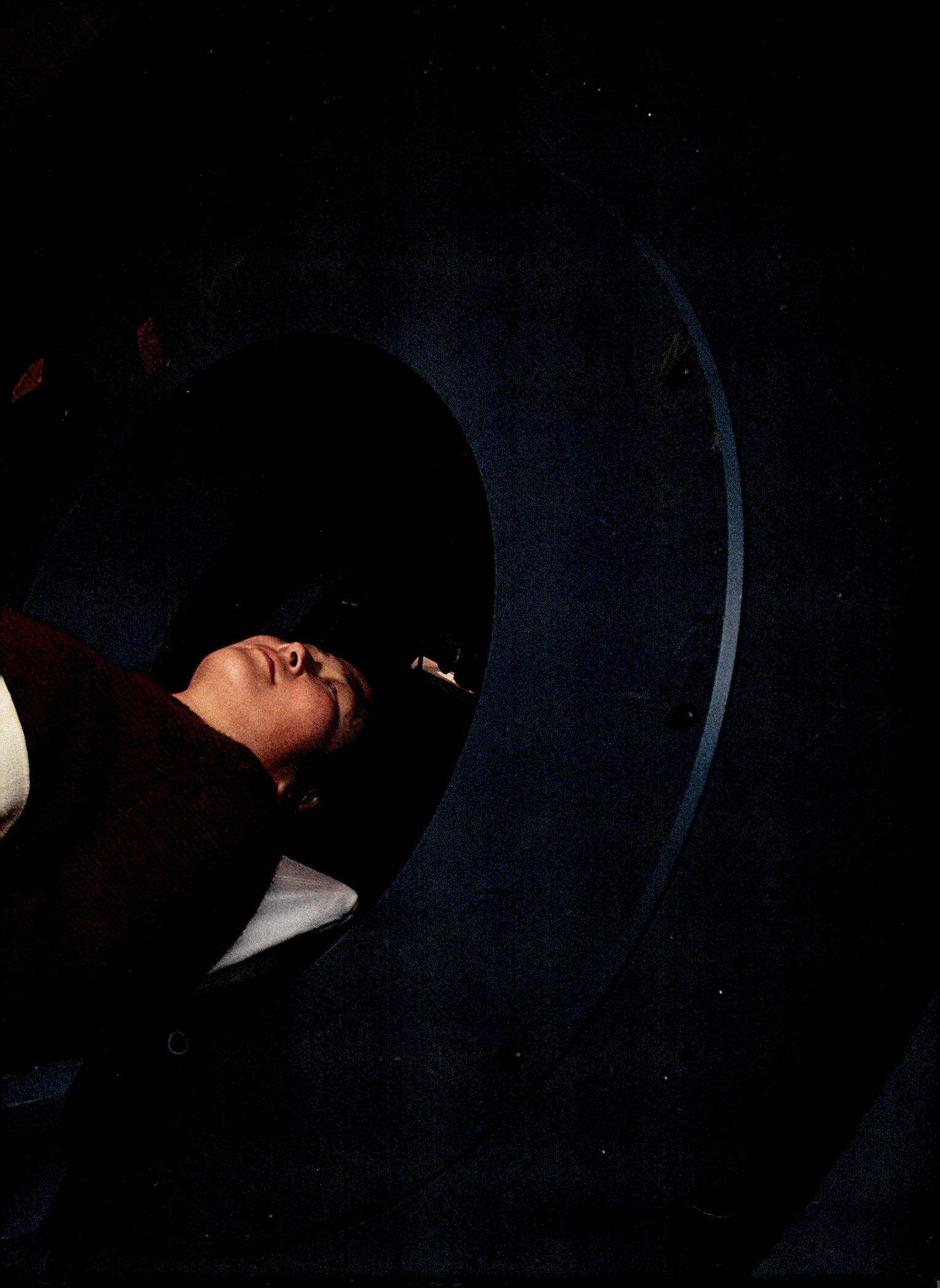

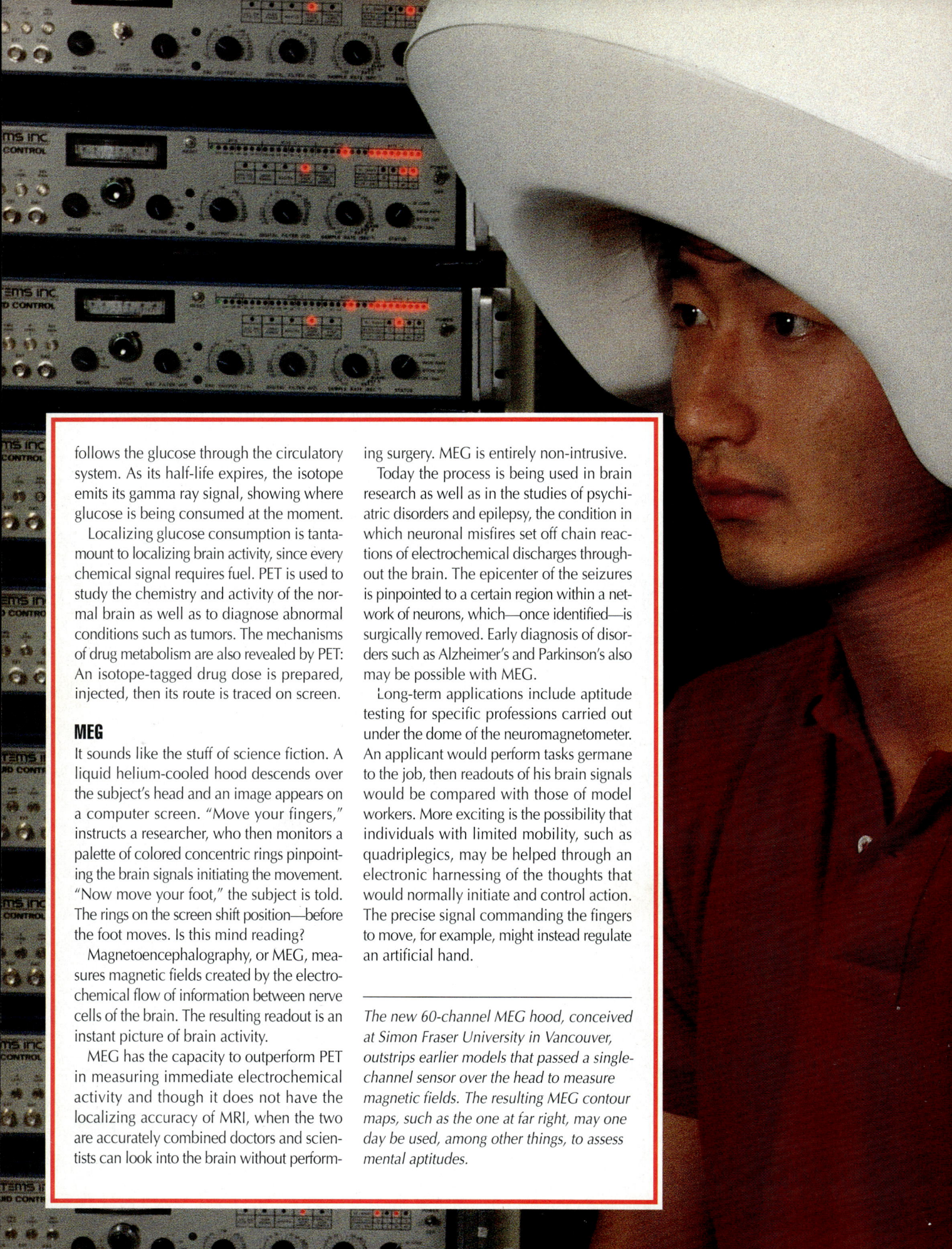

follows the glucose through the circulatory system. As its half-life expires, the isotope emits its gamma ray signal, showing where glucose is being consumed at the moment.

Localizing glucose consumption is tantamount to localizing brain activity, since every chemical signal requires fuel. PET is used to study the chemistry and activity of the normal brain as well as to diagnose abnormal conditions such as tumors. The mechanisms of drug metabolism are also revealed by PET: An isotope-tagged drug dose is prepared, injected, then its route is traced on screen.

MEG

It sounds like the stuff of science fiction. A liquid helium-cooled hood descends over the subject's head and an image appears on a computer screen. "Move your fingers," instructs a researcher, who then monitors a palette of colored concentric rings pinpointing the brain signals initiating the movement. "Now move your foot," the subject is told. The rings on the screen shift position—before the foot moves. Is this mind reading?

Magnetoencephalography, or MEG, measures magnetic fields created by the electrochemical flow of information between nerve cells of the brain. The resulting readout is an instant picture of brain activity.

MEG has the capacity to outperform PET in measuring immediate electrochemical activity and though it does not have the localizing accuracy of MRI, when the two are accurately combined doctors and scientists can look into the brain without performing surgery. MEG is entirely non-intrusive.

Today the process is being used in brain research as well as in the studies of psychiatric disorders and epilepsy, the condition in which neuronal misfires set off chain reactions of electrochemical discharges throughout the brain. The epicenter of the seizures is pinpointed to a certain region within a network of neurons, which—once identified—is surgically removed. Early diagnosis of disorders such as Alzheimer's and Parkinson's also may be possible with MEG.

Long-term applications include aptitude testing for specific professions carried out under the dome of the neuromagnetometer. An applicant would perform tasks germane to the job, then readouts of his brain signals would be compared with those of model workers. More exciting is the possibility that individuals with limited mobility, such as quadriplegics, may be helped through an electronic harnessing of the thoughts that would normally initiate and control action. The precise signal commanding the fingers to move, for example, might instead regulate an artificial hand.

The new 60-channel MEG hood, conceived at Simon Fraser University in Vancouver, outstrips earlier models that passed a single-channel sensor over the head to measure magnetic fields. The resulting MEG contour maps, such as the one at far right, may one day be used, among other things, to assess mental aptitudes.

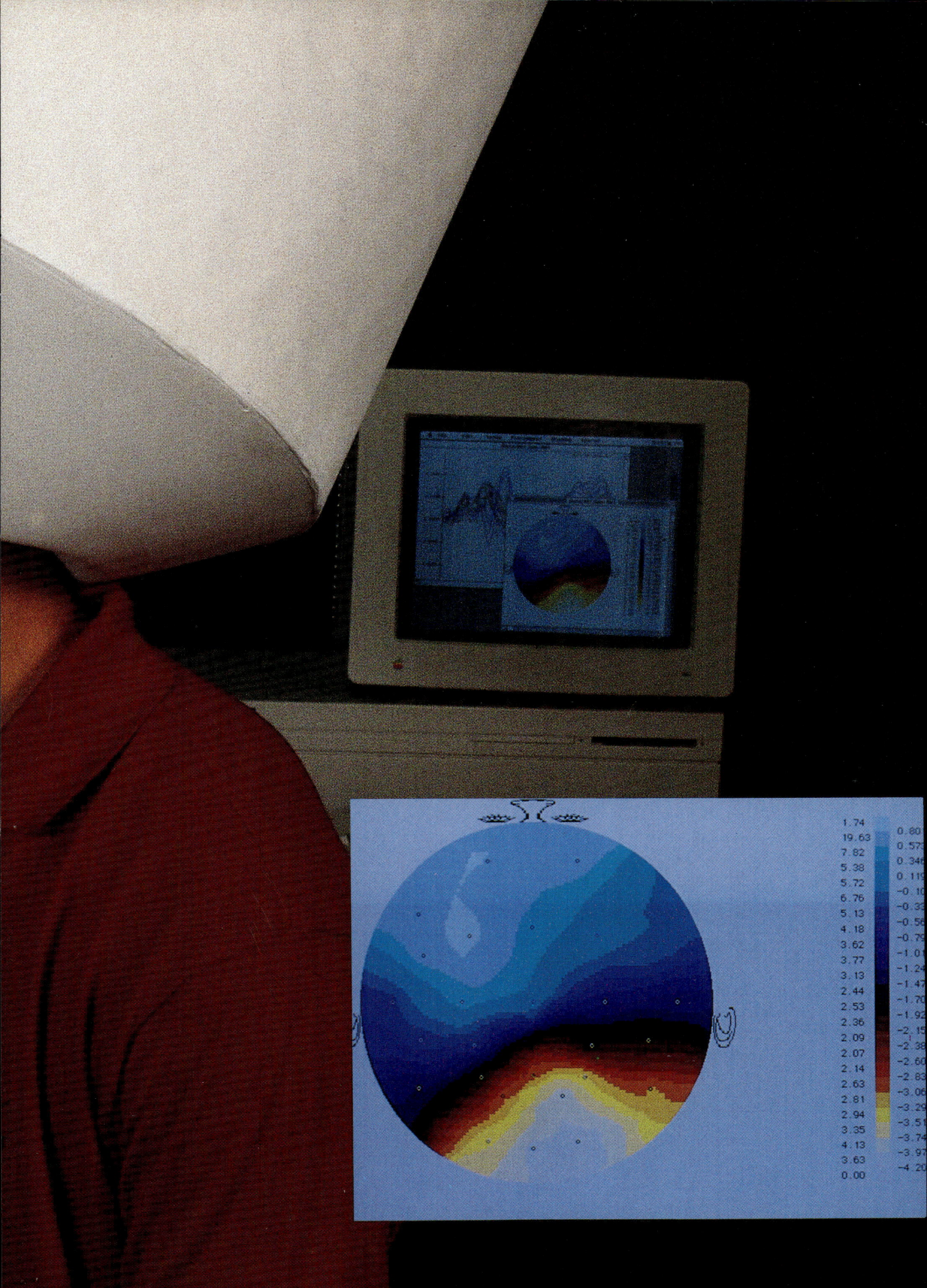

STATES OF MIND

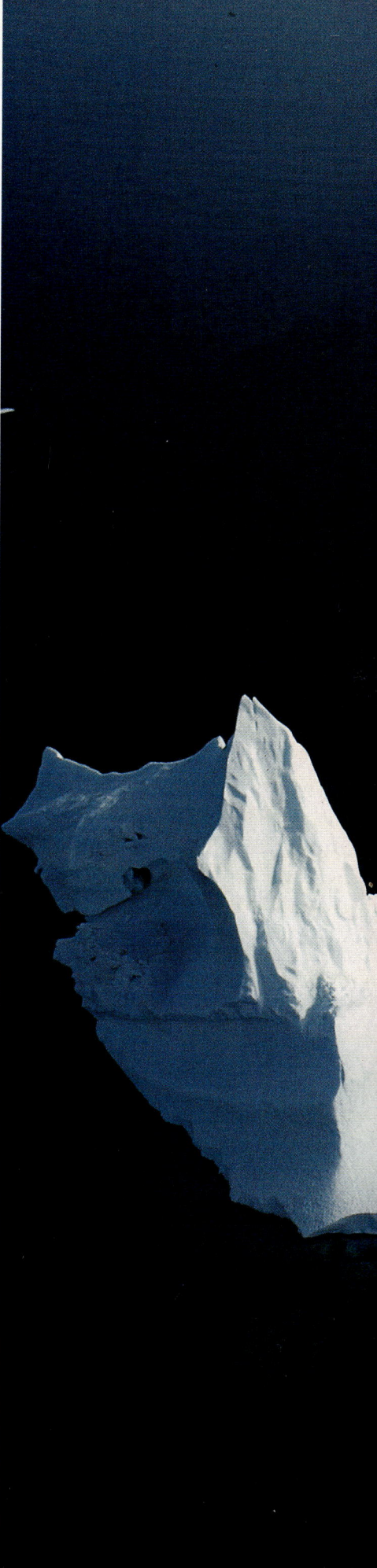

Locked within the brain's deeply furrowed cortex, secure beneath its protective membranes and bony case, lie the wellsprings of memory and dreams, alertness and self-awareness—the conscious and unconscious mind. That bundles of cells, composed of mere matter, are able to produce and direct the nonmaterial panorama of mental life has long confounded philosophers and scientists. Yet any attempt to understand the body's most complicated organ must address this seeming paradox. In medieval times, Christian philosophers resolved the issue by claiming that, while the brain was encased in the body, thoughts and feelings came from God, emanating from a point a few inches above the head. In the 17th Century, the French mathematician and philosopher René Descartes adjusted this hovering entity downward. He argued that man's "rational soul" or "third eye" was centered in the tiny pineal gland that he felt linked the spiritual and physical realms.

Today, neuroscientists have discarded dualism, this theory that the mind is independent of the brain, in favor of monism (from the Greek word *monos*, alone). They place the mind firmly within the physical stuff of the brain and contend that interactions among its billions of neurons produce everything a person mentally experiences. Mind, they contend, is a product of brain activity.

Neurons, humming with activity—networking, processing, interpreting—act with lightning speed on electrochemical information received from inside and outside the body. Incoming messages from the sense organs are routed to various centers in the cortex, the intricate outer layer of the brain. These regions bestow an awareness of the world that constitutes consciousness in its most basic definition. They also stand as doors to the realm beyond awareness, the unconscious.

The brain's curious nocturnal habits, yet another mystery, are now under scrutiny in sleep laboratories around the world. Fitting volunteers with sensors that monitor electrical activity, scientists have given concrete form to the elaborate rhythms

---

Like a floating iceberg, the brain conceals more than it reveals. Consciousness consists of information and stimuli of which the individual is aware. The dark underside of the mind, the unconscious, selectively processes information too trivial—or, perhaps, too frightening—for conscious awareness to deal with.

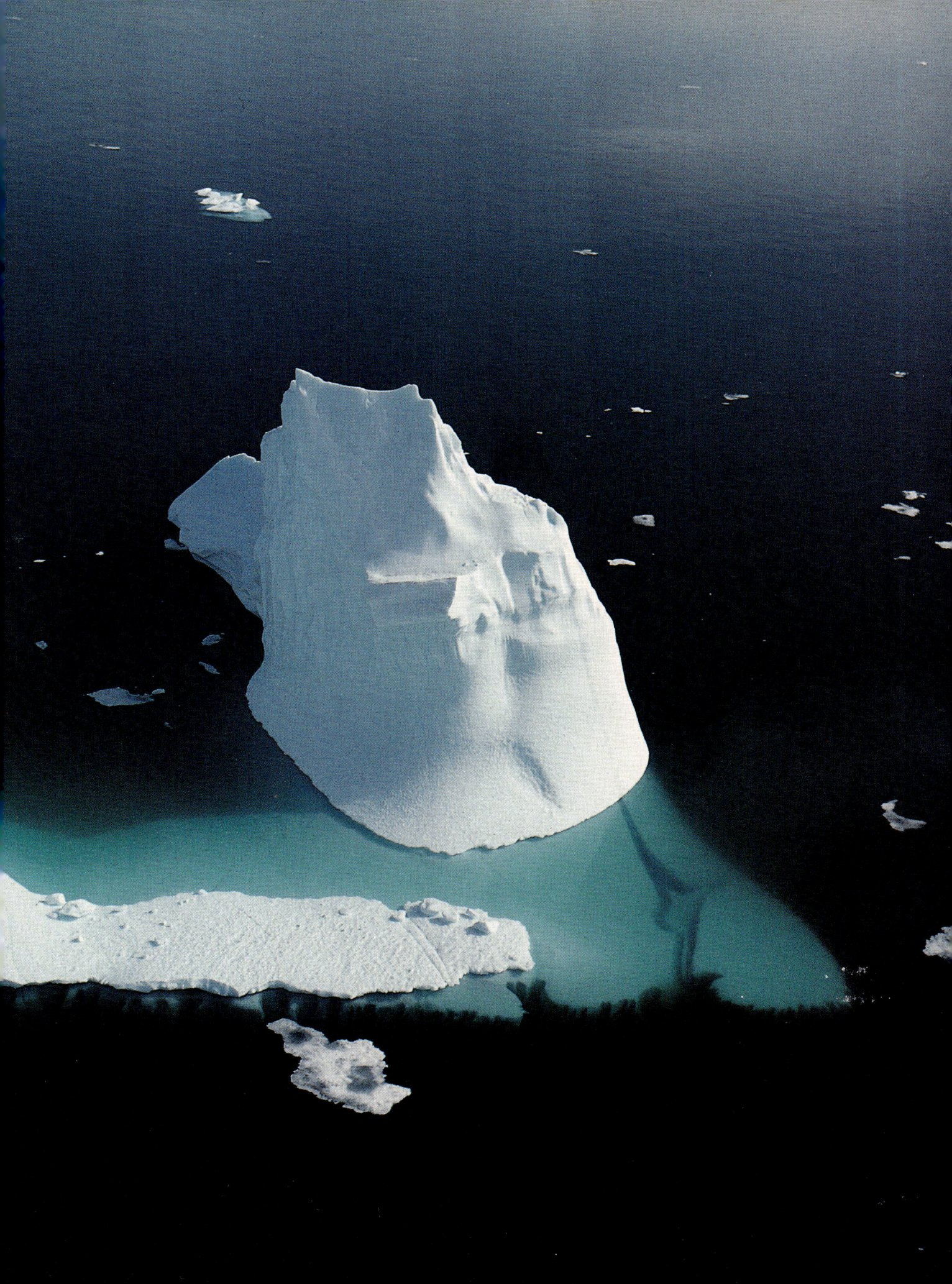

of sleeping and dreaming. Descending into sleep, the brain passes through four distinct phases of varying electrical activity in which the conscious bonds with the rest of the body and the outside world are loosed. Then commences the long, undulating ride toward morning, with its occasional side trips into the land of dreams.

Neuroscientists have probed the boundaries of consciousness by studying people who have undergone surgery or suffered debilitating accidents or strokes where there is localized brain damage resulting from loss of blood flow. They have determined that throughout daily life, the brain processes more information at an unconscious level than at a conscious level, and that the unconscious brain interacts with the conscious brain to guide cognition and behavior. Though this relationship has yet to shed its shroud of obscurity, it is the aim of neuroscientists everywhere to lift the veil.

SCATTERED SIGNALS

In penning the words "Cogito, ergo sum" (I think, therefore I am), René Descartes was making a statement not only about the nature of being, but also about the nature of consciousness. So everpresent is the phenomenon of consciousness that it seems in some respects to constitute life itself.

Consciousness is a multifaceted concept, embracing such seemingly incongruous classes of mental experience as feelings, self-awareness, spatial orientation, language, memory and future planning. Descriptions of consciousness have varied from one era to the next and from one culture to another. Now, contemporary students of the brain—philosophers, linguists, artificial intelligence experts, psychologists, psychiatrists, neurophysicists and neurobiologists—continue the ages-old debate. Broadly speaking, however, the modern neuroscientists of today view consciousness as a product of the brain's activity.

In forming consciousness, the brain synthesizes information funneling in from the outside world, from the body and from specialized subregions of the brain itself, and then formulates a report on the internal and external weather, as it were. Since brain activity is sensitive to the ebb and flow of electrochemical signals, natural daily rhythms and changing conditions outside the body, consciousness must continuously be updated and altered.

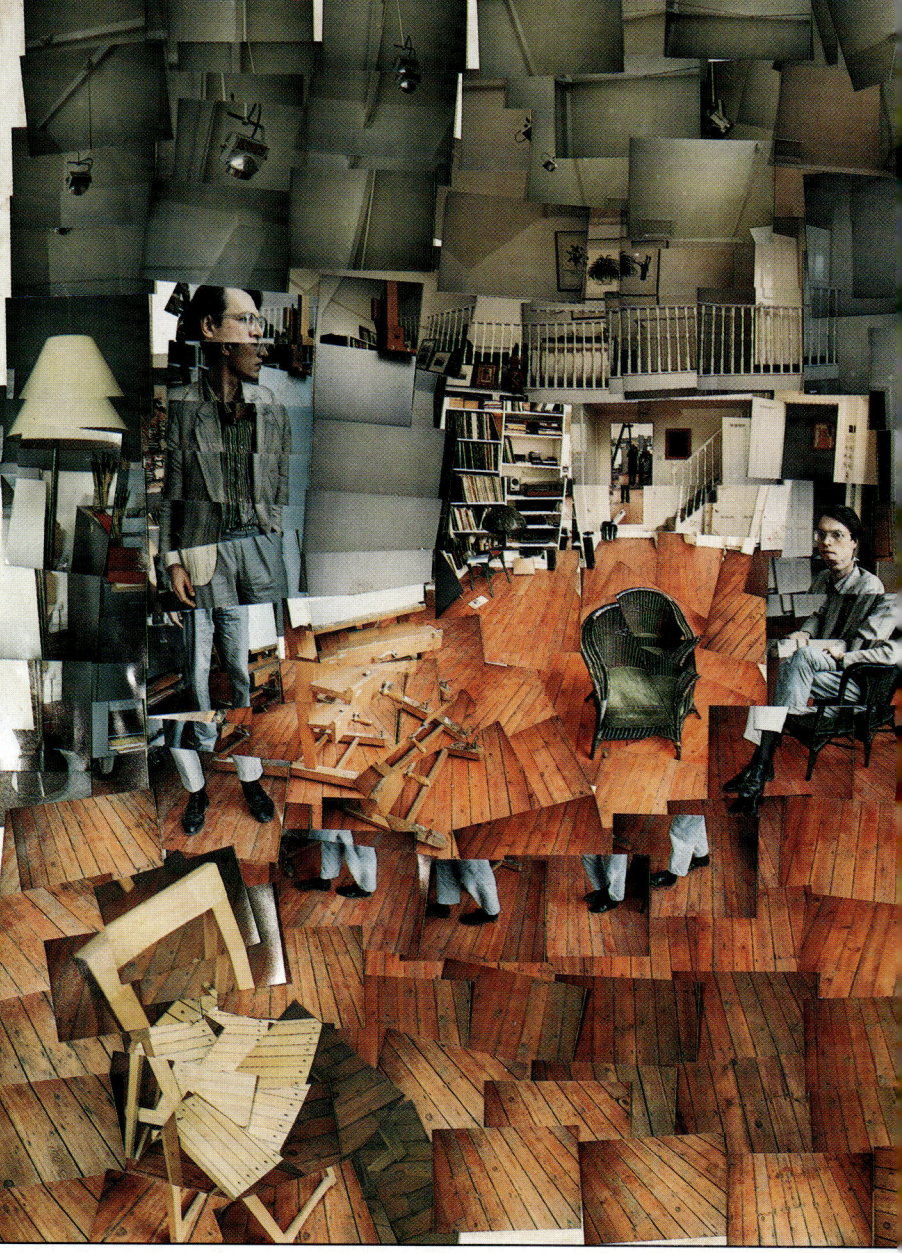

David Hockney's Interior, Pembroke Studios, London, 1972 *is a graphic illustration of the fragmented nature of consciousness. The inner screen of the mind shows a shifting kaleidoscope of incoming stimuli overlaid with memories and colored by emotional associations. The most distinctive feature of consciousness is its disconti-*

By these terms, consciousness is a person's active awareness of his mental and physical state. But consciousness is also selective. The brain heeds some incoming messages and ignores others. This determination of which incoming signals are worthy of being acted upon has been defined as attention, a critical aspect of consciousness. Without it, confusion reigns. The mental illness schizophrenia, characterized by an inability to weed out irrelevant stimuli, is a case in point. In addition to displaying a diminished ability to process signals in some portions of their brains, schizophrenics also have delayed reaction times to stimuli and find it difficult to remain focused.

Researchers have a relatively clear picture of the physical underpinnings of consciousness. Information streaming in from nerve receptors in the skin, muscles, tendons, joints, eyes, ears and mouth passes first through the thalamus and/or the reticular formation—a group of nuclei in the brainstem.

Thus, before even reaching the cortex, impulses have passed through a series of processing regions that behave somewhat like secretaries in an office who screen phone calls, mail and visitors before passing them on to the boss. The reticular formation, sometimes called the ruler of consciousness, stands at the critical junction—both in terms of anatomy and function—of the senses and the higher brain. Vigilant day and night, the neurons of the reticular formation sort all incoming impulses. By some unknown means, they determine which deserve further attention, and having done so, flag important impulses so that the cortex will take note of them. At night, while the cortex is deep in sleep, the reticular formation keeps tabs on the senses and in times of possible danger is first to sound the alarm.

nuity. Yet from the sound and fury of this mental static, the brain manages to fine-tune a remarkably clear, albeit everchanging, conscious focus.

The trunk-like axons of the reticular formation reach upward to connect with the thalamus, a portion of the forebrain composed of two egg-shaped nodules. The thalamus is the second line of processing, and takes a more active role by obtaining information from the reticular formation and some sensory nerves, sending instructions to the muscles, and communicating directly with the cortex. The thalamus also passes on what it has gleaned to the hypothalamus, the tiny, ovoid portion of the forebrain that is the master coordinator of hormones and temperature regulation, as well as hunger and thirst.

Once inside the cortex, which contains three-quarters of the neurons in the brain, incoming signals from the senses are directed to specialized areas. Those from the eyes are routed through the thalamus to a region of the occipital lobe, a portion of the cortex at the back of the brain; those from the ears travel to an area in the temporal lobe. These and other committed areas of the cortex interact with large sections not designated specifically to any one function, called the association cortex. The neural pathways in the association cortex receive information only from within the brain itself and appear to be responsible for most of the brain's highest functions.

One further division in signal processing exists, whereby the brain's right and left halves, or hemispheres, independently take care of incoming sensory inputs from opposite sides of the body. The left side of the body reports to the right hemisphere; the body's right side to the left hemisphere. The hemispheres then share their information through several cable-like bundles of nerve fibers, the largest of which is called the corpus callosum.

Like players in an orchestra, all these brain structures transform the constant influx of signals into the cohesive representation of both inner and outer worlds that is consciousness.

Different states of consciousness have their own characteristic electrical signatures, which scientists can monitor by attaching electrical sensors to the scalp. The readout, called an electroencephalogram (EEG), is created by a stylus tracking along a moving strip of paper, and takes the form of a zigzagging line that gives a real-time representation of electrical activity. The readout produced by the waking brain with the eyes open consists of waves of low amplitude and a mixture of frequencies. When awake—but with eyes closed and the body relaxed—the

MINDWAVES

These mountain-range tracings of EEG readouts show identifiable brainwave patterns that indicate specific states of consciousness. Alert wakefulness (below) is characterized by semi-regular, high-voltage lines at the back of the head (darkest green), progressing to more random, lower-voltage lines near the front of the head (lightest green). When a person becomes drowsy (opposite page), brainwave peaks are shallower and less sharp, indicating a general drop in electrical intensity.

ALERT

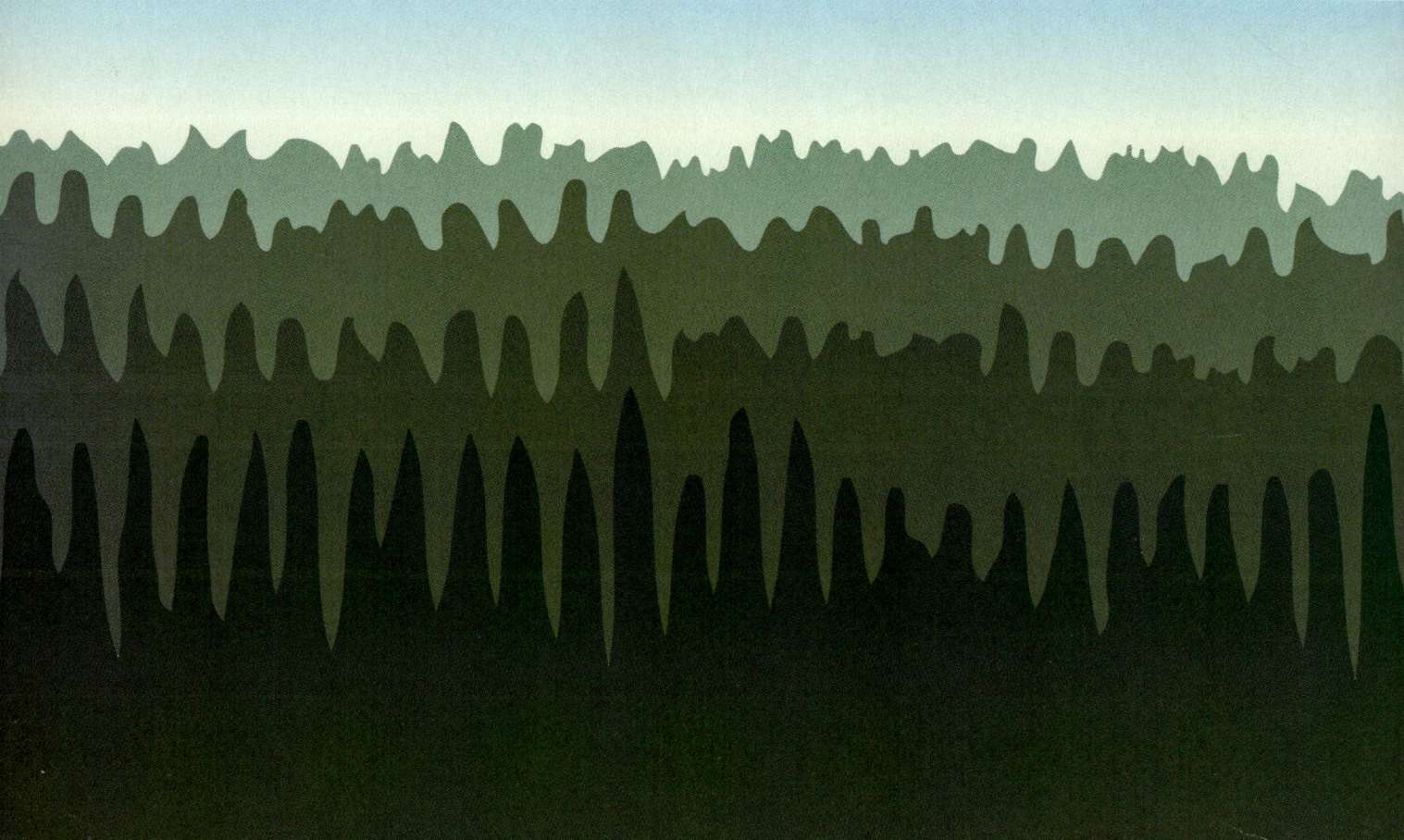

brain produces very regular, rhythmic waves at the rate of between eight and thirteen per second. When sleeping in non-dream sleep stages, the brain yields less rhythmic, slower EEG waves that appear in readouts as a loose, rolling line. When the brain dreams, the waves again are of mixed frequency and create tighter readouts like those produced by the waking brain.

Consciousness, fluctuating by nature, is readily disrupted by drugs or assaults to the cortex such as tumors, strokes or head injuries. Amphetamines, caffeine, tranquilizers and any number of other substances, licit and illicit, can affect electrochemical activity in parts of the brain, thus increasing or diminishing alertness and attention.

In extreme cases, a brain so affected may shut down consciousness temporarily, as in fainting, or on a more prolonged basis, as in coma. Comas may last for days or years, during which the brainstem and hypothalamus, if intact, maintain vital functions. After awakening from coma, some people remain in what is called a persistent vegetative state, in which sleep-wakefulness cycles resume, but perception and awareness—the contents of consciousness—rarely, if ever, return.

Those epileptics who suffer from cortical lesions and have what is called partial complex epilepsy experience temporary losses of awareness, in some cases preceded by visual or auditory hallucinations, unprovoked feelings of fear or anger, loss of speech and other cognitive disturbances. From dramatic experiments with people who had undergone surgical treatment for epilepsy came the revelation that consciousness is underlain by another sort of brain activity that cannot be directly reached, unconsciousness.

In the 1950s, researchers Michael Gazzaniga and Roger Sperry at the California Institute of Technology, studied a group of individuals in whom the corpus cal-

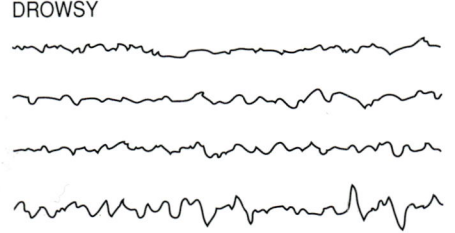

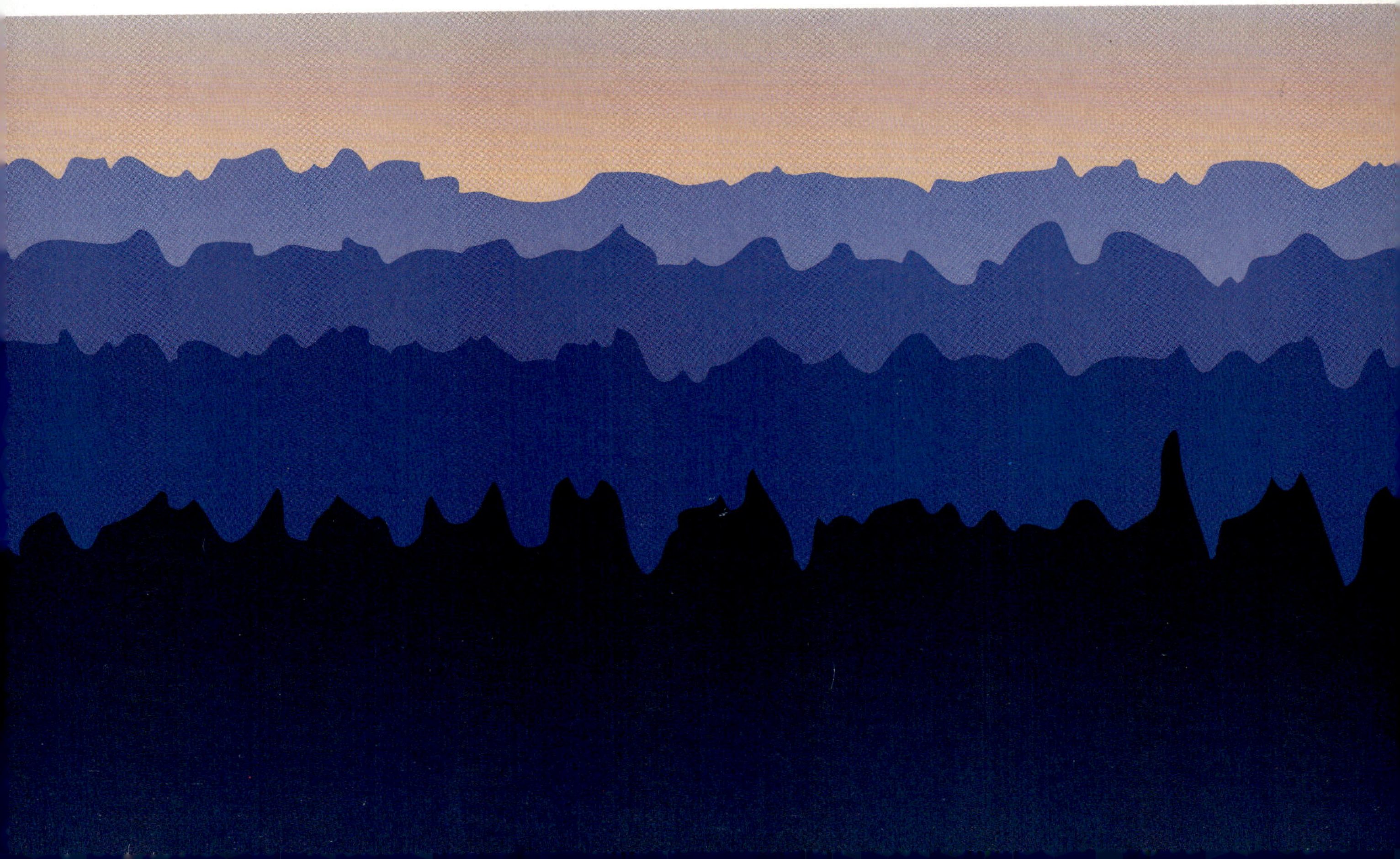

DROWSY

losum had been cut in an operation designed to stop uncontrollable epileptic attacks. Severing the cable of communication between the brain's halves, Gazzaniga and Sperry discovered, had created patients whose left hands literally did not know what their right hands were doing *(page 122)*.

Studies of other so-called split-brain patients, conducted in the 1970s by Gazzaniga, have revealed that the left side of the brain will struggle to explain behavior that has been prompted by commands directed to the right brain. One subject whose right brain was given the command "Walk" did get up and cross the room. However, when asked what he was doing, he answered that he was going to get a soda and was entirely unaware of the real reason for his action.

In the early part of this century, Sigmund Freud postulated the existence of the unconscious, among other things the repository of sexual or violent urges too overwhelming to be dealt with in raw form. To Freud, these repressed wishes fed into waking life, creating psychological disorders. But studies like those performed by Gazzaniga and Sperry have challenged Freud's views.

Freud's supposed repression mechanism may, in fact, be built into the very structure of the brain. Certain nonverbal aspects of awareness—beliefs, desires and memories—may be laid down in such a way that they are only indirectly available to the left brain. In fact, any information that is highly charged emotionally may be processed and stored by the unconscious brain before even reaching the consciousness. If the brain does employ such biological "black box" technology, some emotional content that shapes personality may ever remain unreachable.

In the 1973 movie The Exorcist, *the image of a ghoulish face flashes on the screen in the middle of a dream sequence for two frames or one-twelfth of a second—too fast for most viewers' conscious perception, but long enough to heighten the tension. Experiments using electrodes reveal the brain responds to stimuli that remain at the unconscious level. Although subliminal messages have been banned from television advertising, it is not certain that they are capable of influencing behavior.*

SLEEPYHEAD

Poets and artists have likened the journey from wakefulness into sleep to the more profound transition from life into death. Humans asleep were seen to surrender conscious control and pass into a netherworld, apparently devoid of volition and emotions, ensnared in a death-like immobility.

This linking of sleep and death influenced scientific thinking even into the early part of the 20th Century. During sleep, it was held, the hurly-burly of awareness ceased and the brain lapsed into leaden torpor. In 1913, the French scientist Henri Pieron argued that sleep temporarily but completely severed the brain's ties with the sensory organs and the motor neurons responsible for muscle control. Pieron believed this cleavage from the external world was vital: It was the body's way of giving the brain a much-needed rest. Further elaboration of this theory in the 1930s led some researchers to cast the issue in terms of stimulation thresholds. If the brain were bombarded with sufficient stimuli, it would remain alert; otherwise, it would sink inexorably into sleep.

But already, a substantially different portrait of the sleeping brain had begun to emerge, and in 1951, a graduate student at the University of Chicago made an observation that provoked a radical shift in understanding. While studying sleeping infants, Eugene Aserinsky noticed that at various times during the night, the infants' eyes would flutter back and forth under their closed lids. Aserinsky reported this finding to his professor, Nathaniel Kleitman, who was intrigued enough to undertake further studies. Kleitman set up a laboratory where subjects could be watched and monitored simultaneously by electroencephalograph, and he began mustering volunteers for his experiments.

STATES OF MIND

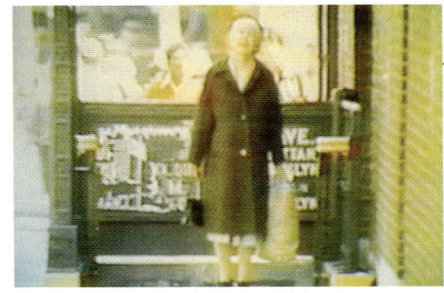
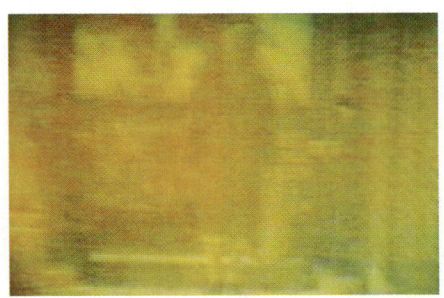
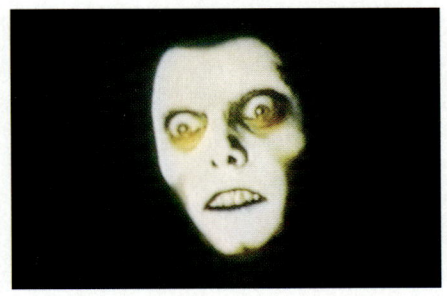

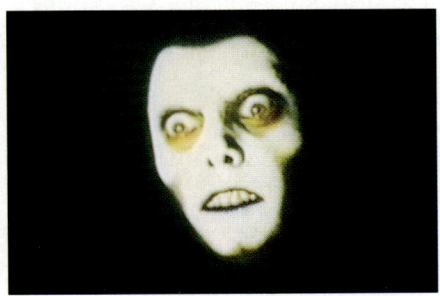
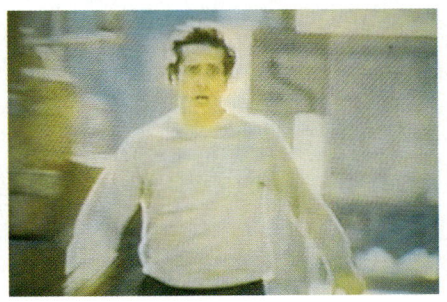

Two years later he announced that adults also displayed periods of so-called rapid eye movements, or REM. Not only that, REM sleep coincided with a speeding up of heartbeat, breathing and the frequency of brain waves. Kleitman went on, with medical student William Dement, to describe the brain's alternation between two distinct types of sleep, REM and non-REM, each with its own set of physiological accompaniments.

Clearly, sleep, far from a retreat into passivity, is a time of ongoing neuronal bustle punctuated by flurries of excitation rivaling those that take place in the alert brain. Scientists can now chart in detail a typical night's sleep of seven to eight hours in duration, as shown on page 60.

Contrary to popular belief, the body does not so much drift into sleep as switch into it, as evidenced by a sharp change in the wave pattern produced on an EEG readout over a minute or so. Having reduced its perception of and response to peripheral inputs, the brain moves through four progressively deeper stages during which the low-voltage alpha waves of the waking brain give way to theta, and delta waves, which occur at more protracted intervals and carry greater energy.

During Stage 1 sleep, the EEG signal shifts from mainly alpha waves to mainly theta, while the would-be sleeper may experience an array of near-hallucinations. As thoughts wander and scattered images and sounds flit through the semiconsciousness, brain waves continue to slow. Muscle tone diminishes. Now and again, for no more than a second or so, the mainly theta waves of what is now Stage 2 sleep leap upward in small, fast bursts called spindles—volleys of rhythmic beta frequency waves—and K complexes—sharp upward waves followed immediately by steep downward ones. The brain begins to move into Stages 3 and 4 where very slow delta waves dominate the EEG trace. Young adults spend roughly 50 percent of the night in Stage 2 sleep; about 25 percent in Stages 3 and 4.

About 20 minutes into the night, when a healthy young adult has plunged into the slow wave, or delta, sleep of Stages 3 and 4, the heart rate has dampened, blood pressure has declined, the intestines and muscles have relaxed. The sleeper has reached the deepest point of non-REM sleep and can be aroused only with difficulty. Then the brain's tempo picks up again and suddenly, about 90 minutes into the night, shifts into high gear. Faster, lower amplitude waves intermixed with beta activity appear on the EEG, mimicking the pattern generated by the waking brain. This is REM sleep, and it is accompanied and defined by three distinct physical alterations: relatively low voltage, mixed frequency EEG; rapid eye movements; and the absence of voluntary muscle tone.

The first episode of REM lasts only three to ten minutes in young adults and is followed at roughly 90-minute intervals by three or four more bouts, which progressively grow in duration across the night. The last REM period of the night may last 45 minutes or so. Dreams are reported more than 80 percent of the time when sleepers are awakened from REM sleep. Vivid, illogical flights of fantasy fill the REM-sleep landscape. Sleepers awakened from non-REM sleep report dreams 20 to 30 percent of the time, though in this state the mind's output is more plodding and straightforward, mulling over ideas or events of the day.

Precisely how the brain initiates and coordinates the process of sleep remains a mystery. Evidence suggests that the key neurons lie in several structures within the brainstem and hypothalamus.

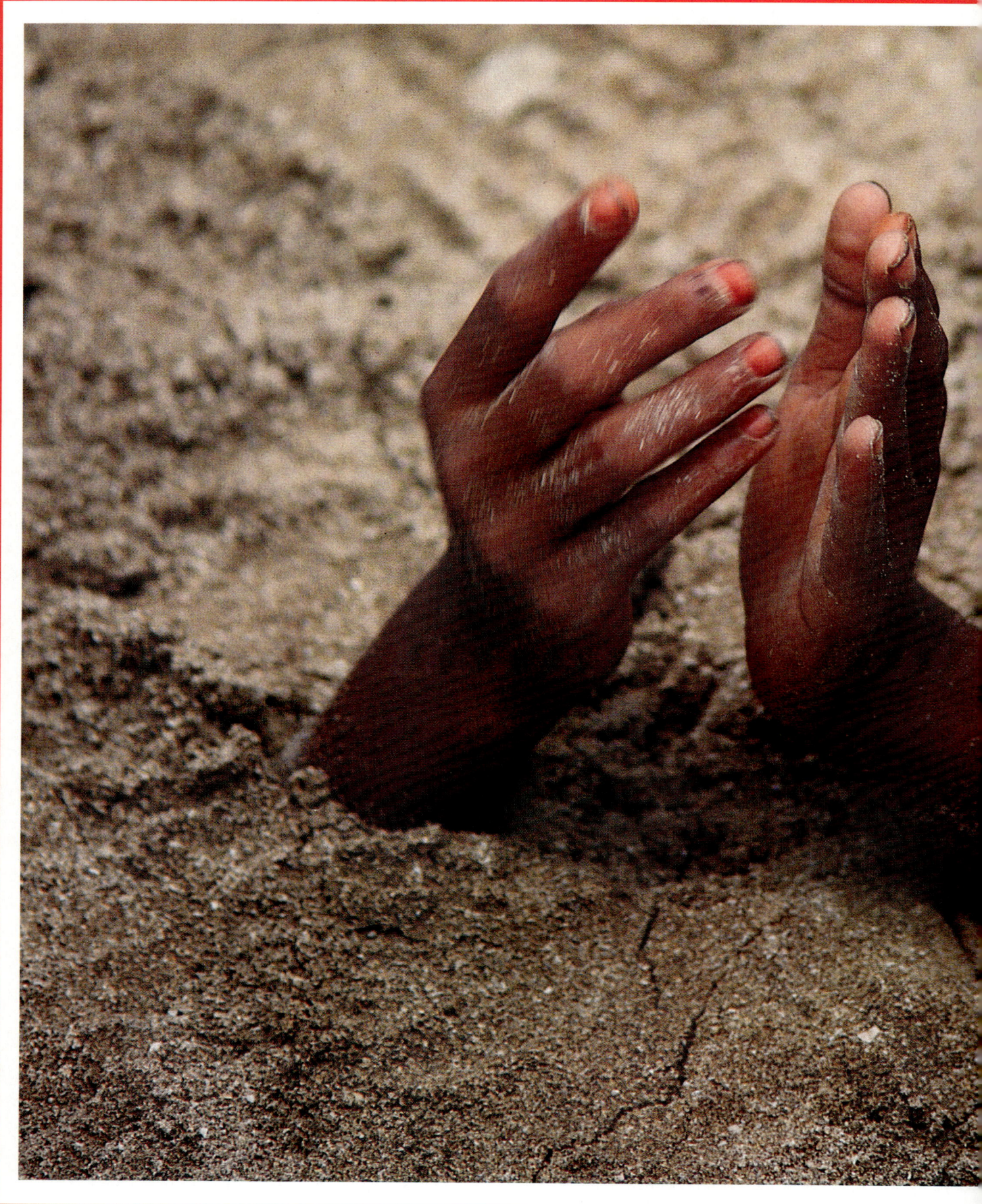

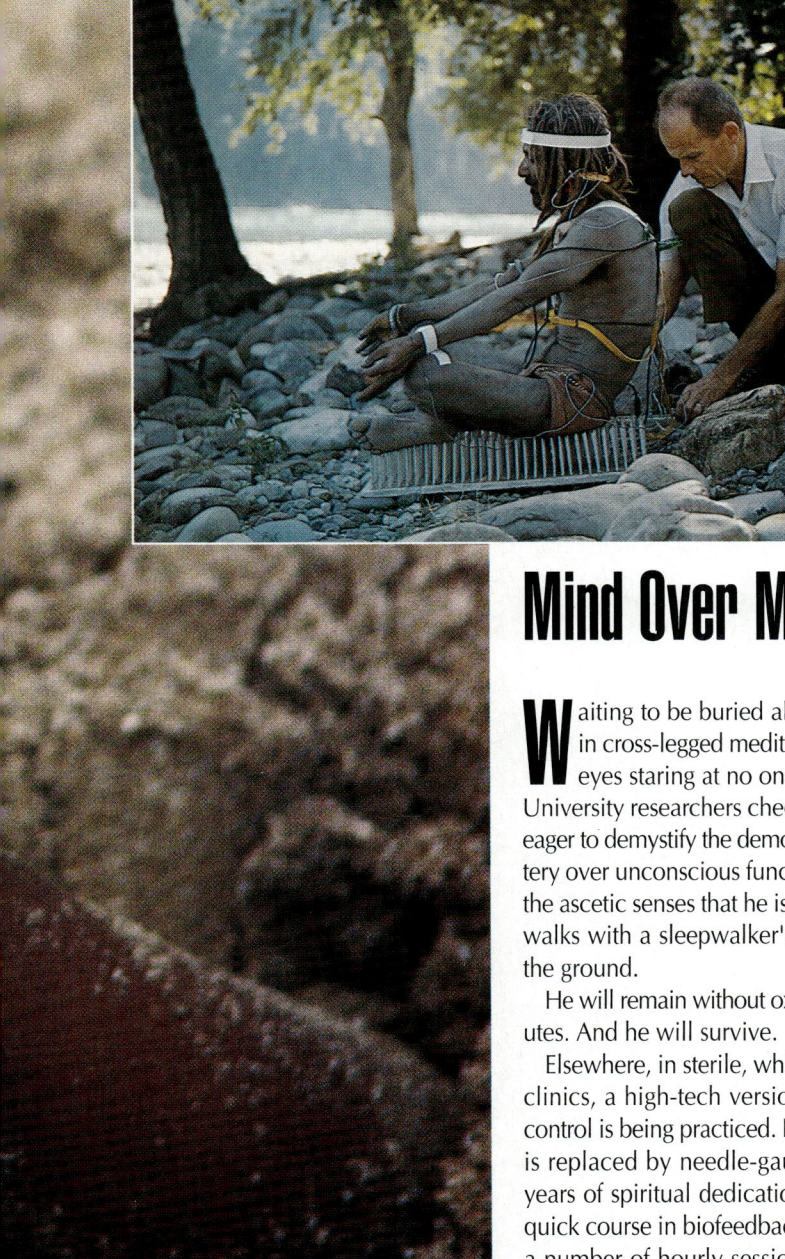

Technology meets spirituality as a yogi is equipped with electrodes to measure his physical responses while sitting on a bed of nails.

Mind Over Matter

Waiting to be buried alive, the yogi sits in cross-legged meditation, half-lidded eyes staring at no one definable spot. University researchers check their watches, eager to demystify the demonstration of mastery over unconscious functions. Eventually the ascetic senses that he is ready, rises, and walks with a sleepwalker's gait to a pit in the ground.

He will remain without oxygen for 45 minutes. And he will survive.

Elsewhere, in sterile, white psychological clinics, a high-tech version of mind-body control is being practiced. Esoteric mystique is replaced by needle-gauge clarity here, years of spiritual dedication obviated by a quick course in biofeedback technology. In a number of hourly sessions, subjects will have learned to regulate blood flow to their hands and feet, slow or speed up heart rate—and even to alter brainwaves.

In both settings individuals monitor and control physiological processes through an acquired sensitivity to data normally privy only to the unconscious brain. Biofeedback uses green monitor blips and siren-like whines to report the same information that nerves feed to brain centers such as the hypothalamus, medulla oblongata and the somatosensory cortex—or, in the case of brainwaves, information originating in the thalamus itself.

Using EEG to tune in alpha waves or a modulating tone to signal blood heat is analogous to relying on the eyes to aim for a bull's-eye; buried alive or resting comfortably on sharp nails, the unwired yogi manages the same feat through meditation alone.

Buried alive with his praying hands toward heaven, an Indian yogi is in a trance-like state that reduces his requirement for oxygen.

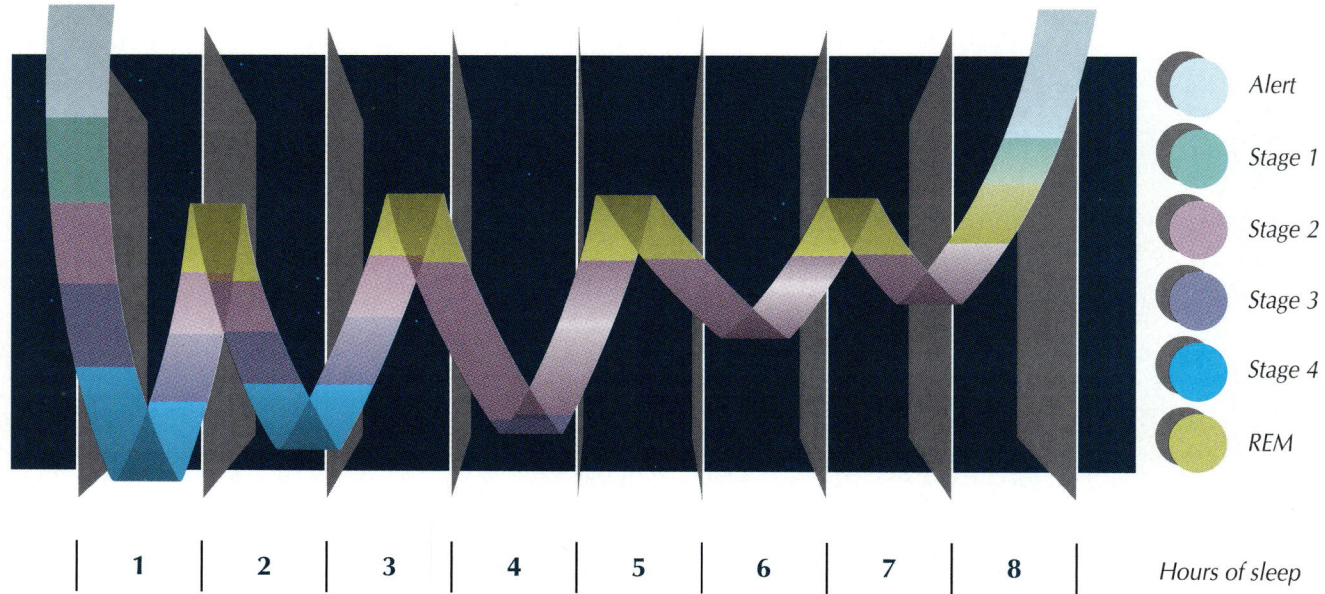

CHARTING A NIGHT'S SLEEP
Roughly every 90 minutes the brain guides the sleeper through a valley in the land of Nod. The deepest descent occurs early in the night; as morning approaches, longer and longer periods are spent in the fantastical landscape of REM.

The brainstem, at the back of the brain, sends bundles of nerves down into the spine. These serve as conduits for messages traveling in from the senses and out from the higher brain to the muscles. In this way, the brainstem is a pathway to consciousness. Above it, nestled at the base of the cerebrum, is the hypothalamus. Both the brainstem and the hypothalamus contain divisions that mediate sleep.

The hypothalamus, as a master regulator of hormones, relegates separate tasks to its divisions, and it seems that its preoptic area is involved in temperature control while the suprachiasmatic nucleus acts as a pacemaker for circadian rhythms, the roughly 24-hour-long cycles that shape an assortment of bodily processes, including waking and sleeping.

Like all neurons, those in the brainstem and hypothalamus communicate by neurotransmitters. Released into the synapses between neurons, neurotransmitters stimulate or dampen neuronal activity, each producing a different effect. Bundles of nerve cell bodies in the brainstem's specialized areas—the raphe nuclei and the locus coeruleus—employ serotonin and noradrenaline respectively. Levels of both these chemicals, as well as a third transmitter, acetylcholine, seem to be involved in regulating sleep.

The control of sleep is exerted over a diffuse network—or networks—of neurons spreading throughout the brainstem and hypothalamus and into the thicket of nerves contained in the reticular formation, a key processor of signals speeding in from the senses. This dense network is thought to selectively direct the firing of serotonin and noradrenaline neurons to turn REM on and off.

The non-REM–REM patterns of sleep itself are subsumed in the larger cycle of the circadian rhythm, which under normal circumstances unfolds over the course of 24 hours. From waking through sleeping to waking again, the body undergoes a carefully plotted transit. Temperature fluctuates about two to three degrees, reaching its zenith in the afternoon and its nadir from two to five in the morning. Hormones are formed and released, urine is produced and excreted, appetite triggered, all in pace with an internal clock calibrated with cues from the environment.

Time-lapse photography, such as the series opposite, sheds light on the mysteries of both normal and disordered sleep. Veteran insomniacs who regularly "don't sleep a wink all night" often awaken at sleep clinics to the photographic evidence that their sleep is sound. Because thinking continues during non-REM stages, sleepers can convince themselves they are awake.

Almost all other organisms exhibit circadian rhythms, from morning glories, which bloom with strict regularity regardless of the presence or absence of light, to minute golden-brown algae, which live buried in beach sand when the tides are high, but move to the surface when the ocean ebbs and the sun is up. The actions of these plants and animals are dictated by biological clocks that are responsive to external stimuli.

Among birds and most mammals, the light-sensitive pineal gland acts as the pacemaker, triggering the release of the hormone melatonin in response to darkness. In humans, the chief pacemakers appear to be the suprachiasmatic nuclei found on either side of the hypothalamus, which receive inputs directly from the eyes. Sunlight, entering the eyes and translated into signals feeding into the suprachiasmatic nuclei, seems to serve the vital purpose of training the body's rhythms to the 24-hour solar day. However, other habits such as work, meals and social schedules may reinforce this effect.

Scientists believe that such nonbiological time cues actually sway our biological routines. When experimental volunteers have been isolated in windowless rooms and deprived of clocks and all environmental cues they have consistently settled into circadian cycles lasting about 25 hours, a period closer to the lunar than the solar day. A few people go through a phase in which their days become desynchronized. For them, a "day" can be as long as 53 hours, or as short as 19, though some circadian biological rhythms continue to follow a 25-hour cycle. Their body temperature, say, might peak twice in a 50-hour "day."

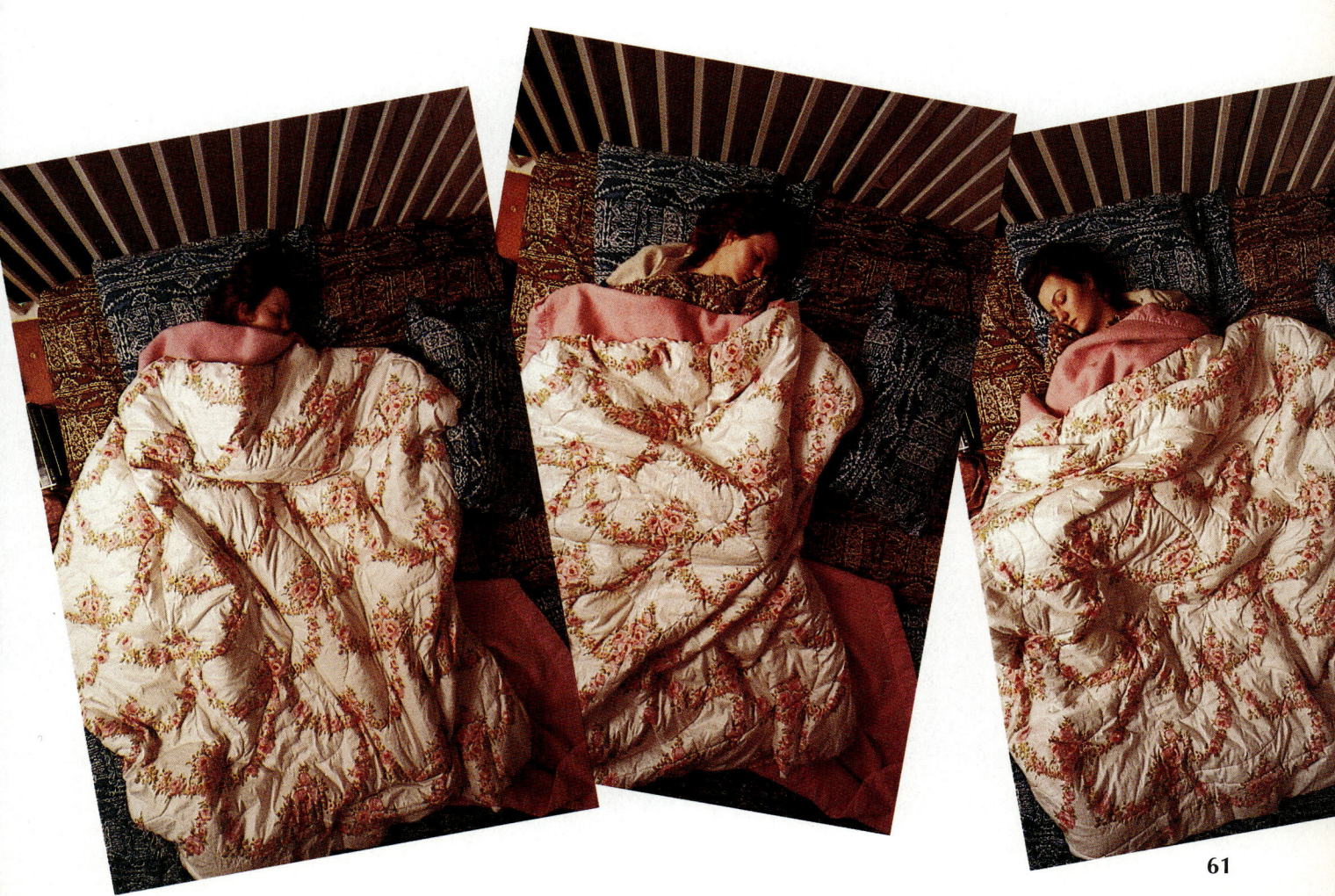

If humans display versatility in being able to synchronize their rhythms according to solar and societal variables, they also display at least one major, inflexible trait: They seem to be programmed to sleep at night. Forced to sleep by day and work at night, people almost always develop the hallmark symptoms of physiological stress. Shift workers may eventually develop a tolerance for late-night stints, but most complain of persistent fatigue and experience difficulties with their moods, digestion and alertness. Often, even though they go to bed exhausted after duty on the swing (4 p.m. to midnight) or graveyard (midnight to 8 a.m.) shift, they suffer from insomnia.

Studies have confirmed that efficiency plummets among workers who are shunted between swing and graveyard shifts with frequency. The Three Mile Island nuclear accident in Harrisburg, Pennsylvania, happened under the watch of a crew that had been rotated in this manner, as did the fiascos at the Chernobyl nuclear plant in the Soviet Union and the Union Carbide chemical plant in Bhopal, India. The pattern has cropped up at airports as well, where near misses due to slip-ups by oft-rotated air traffic controllers proliferate at night. In addition, airline crews also must cope with jet lag, which delivers another blow to the biological clock. Jumping between time zones scrambles the body rhythms and it can take days for them to restabilize *(page 64)*.

Scientists are uncertain why nighttime sleep has been hardwired into the brain. Perhaps there are evolutionary reasons. Millions of years ago, survival may have

Only in the REM stage, when limb muscles are paralyzed, does a person sleep "like a log." Captured on film at 15-minute intervals, a slumbering test subject tosses and turns the night away, moving from one sleep stage to another. During the 45-minute period of the second, third and fourth photos of this sequence, the sleeper lies motionless in REM dreamland. Switching into non-REM sleep, she rolls over and changes position.

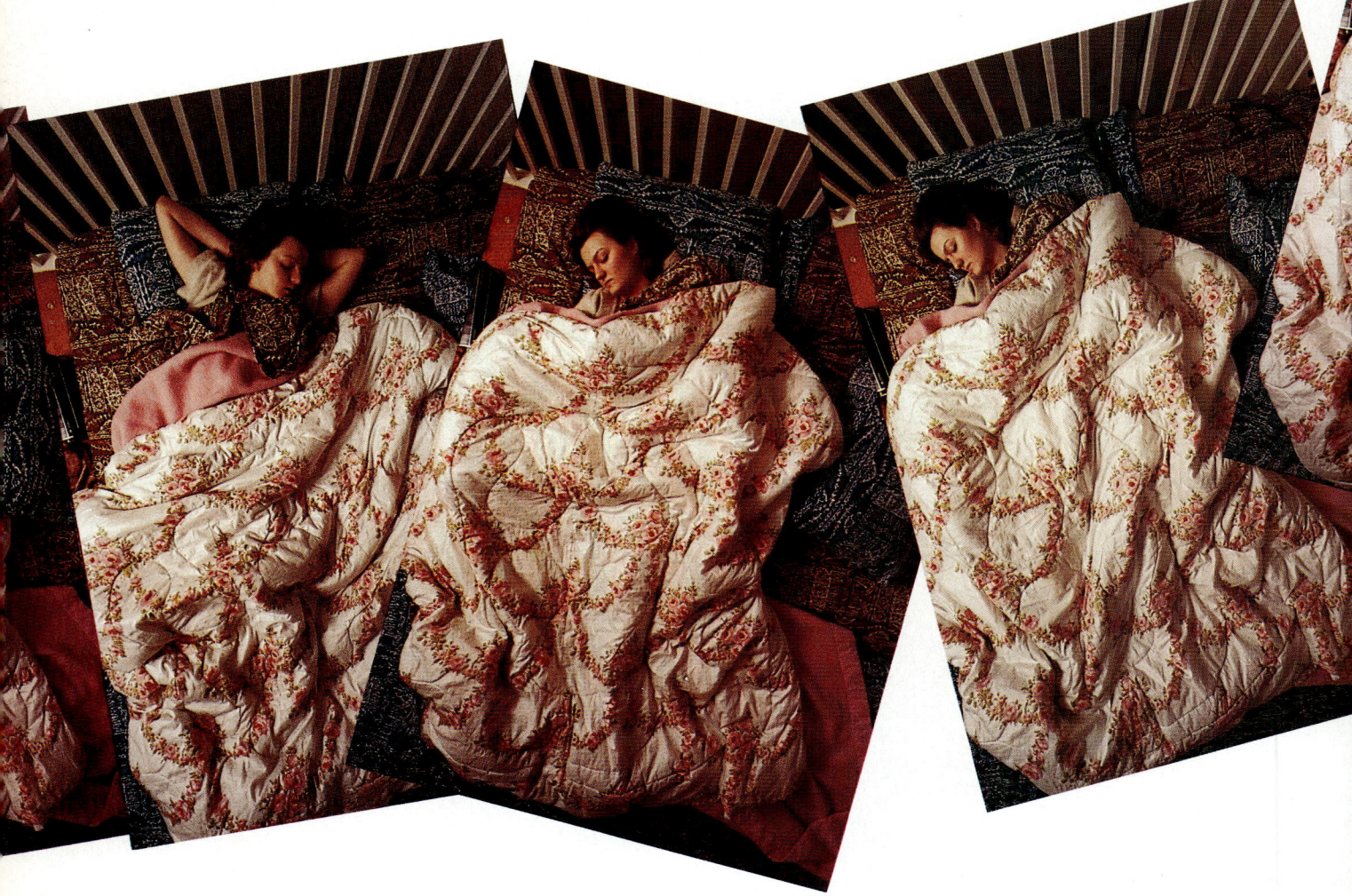

depended on hunting by day and retreating to caves at night to avoid other predators. This may also explain a secondary circadian rhythm that causes people to become drowsy in midafternoon. Napping for a few hours after lunch may have arisen originally as an adaptive strategy. Perhaps the midday heat on the African savannas drove *Homo sapiens* to find a patch of shade for a place to rest and to conserve energy and liquids. In any case, napping for a few hours at midafternoon increases alertness and improves mood during the rest of the day.

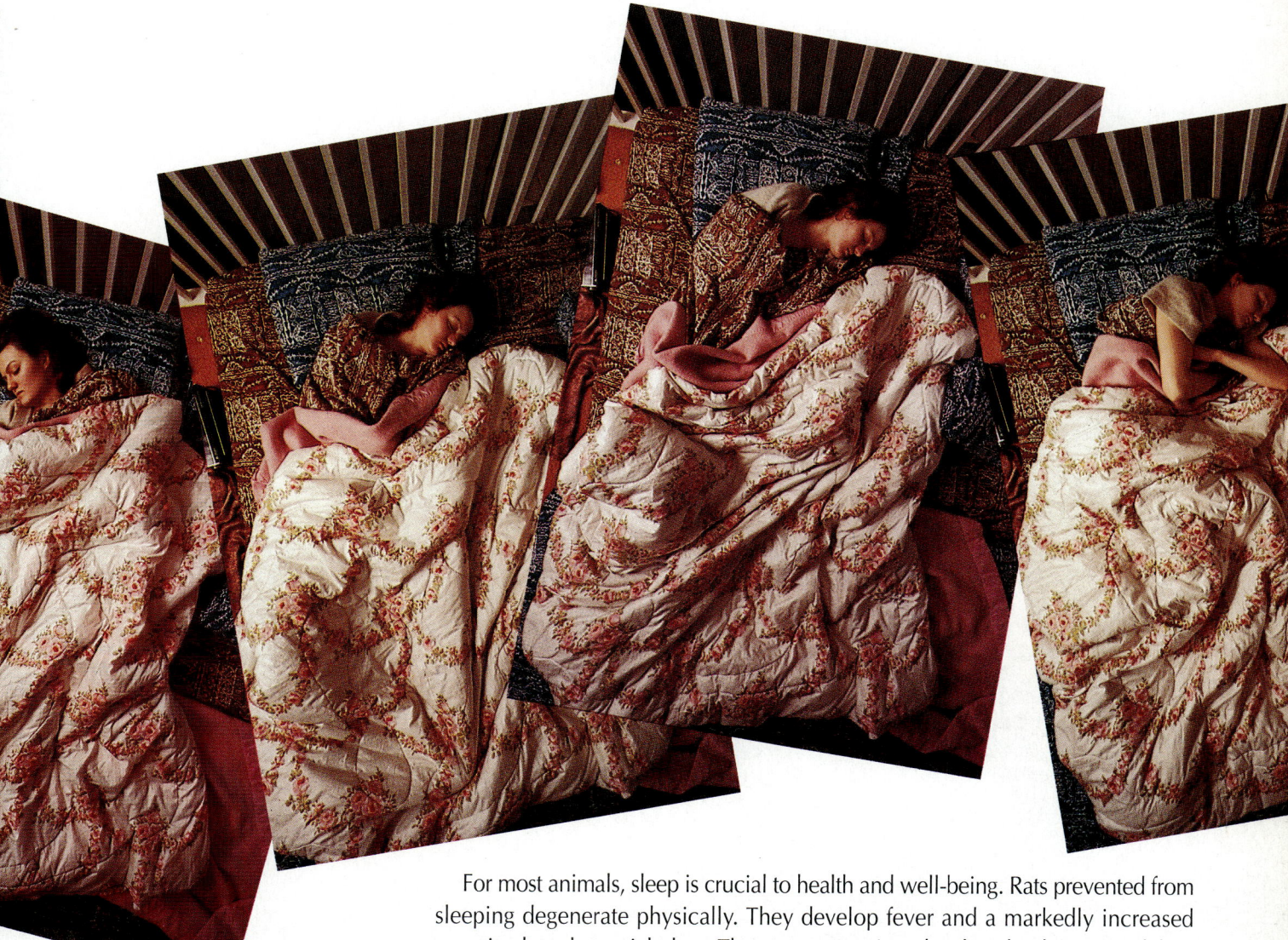

For most animals, sleep is crucial to health and well-being. Rats prevented from sleeping degenerate physically. They develop fever and a markedly increased appetite, but also weight loss. They stop grooming, develop skin lesions and then suffer lower temperatures and, ultimately, die. Humans also need sleep, although requirements vary from person to person. Some people get by on as little as three or four hours' sleep a night, some cannot do with less than twelve or fourteen; however the vast majority need from six to eight and a half hours—defined as the normal range—with the amount diminishing slightly as they age.

The ancient Greeks held that during sleep, Asclepius, the god of medicine, cured the body of its ills. Echoing this belief, Shakespeare wrote that sleep "knits up the ravell'd sleave of care." Indeed, scientists have found that hormones released during the night promote cellular mending and tissue repair, thus acting

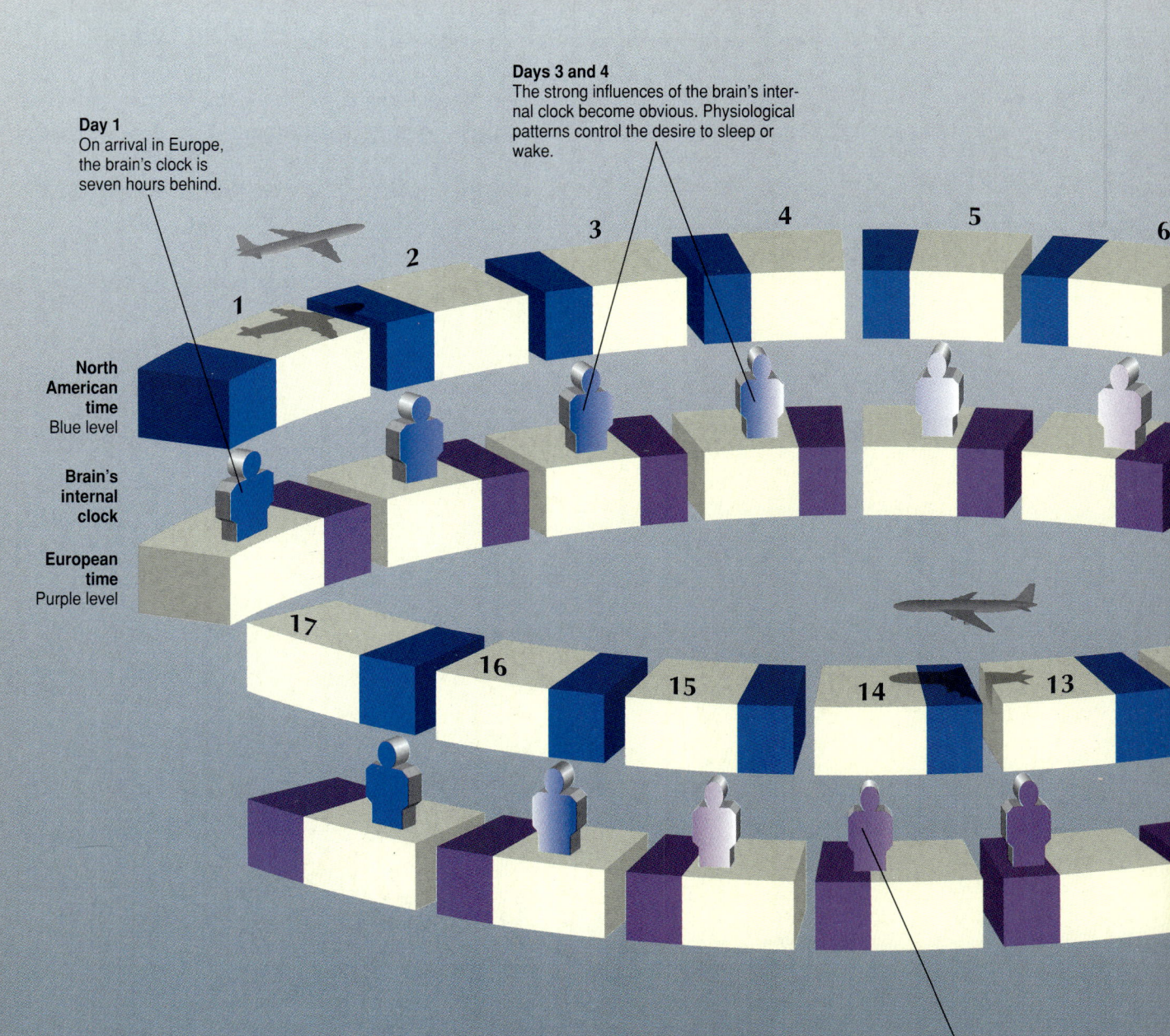

Day 1
On arrival in Europe, the brain's clock is seven hours behind.

Days 3 and 4
The strong influences of the brain's internal clock become obvious. Physiological patterns control the desire to sleep or wake.

North American time
Blue level

Brain's internal clock

European time
Purple level

Day 14
Though it is easier for the brain to turn back its clock, the traveler still experiences a few days of crankiness and somnolence at home.

BODY CLOCK BLUES
This chart illustrates jet lag experienced by a traveler going from North America to Europe and back over a 17-day period. The top level represents the nights (blue) and days (white) according to the time in North America. The bottom level represents the nights (purple) and days (white) according to the time in Europe. The silhouette figure between the two levels shows the changes in the traveler's biological clock. As he arrives in Europe the body clock is set for North American night, so he appears as blue (North American night) in the white (daytime) of Europe. As the days pass, his body clock slowly adjusts to clock time in Europe until he is in sync (purple on purple block of night 11). As the jet-setter heads home, desynchronization takes place again until full resynchronization is achieved (blue figure under the blue block of night 17).

STATES OF MIND

Time Flies

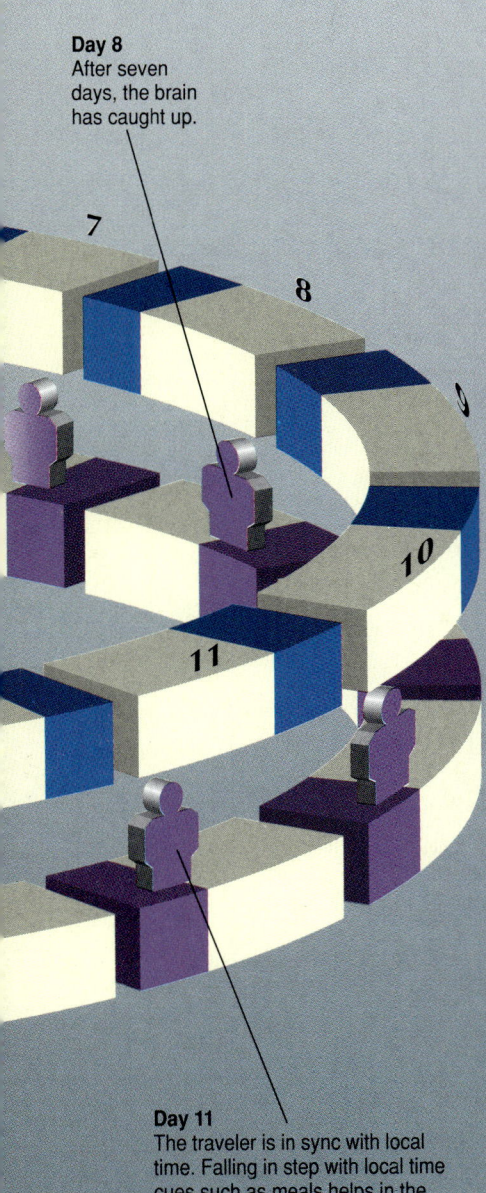

Day 8
After seven days, the brain has caught up.

Day 11
The traveler is in sync with local time. Falling in step with local time cues such as meals helps in the adjustment process.

A transatlantic flight arrives in Athens from New York at 6 a.m., early enough to pass through customs, stow bags in a hotel and still have a jump on a full day of sightseeing. Except for one hitch: A little 10,000-neuron clock within the traveler's brain insists it is not early morning but bedtime.

By noon Athens-time it is hard to keep from nodding off—no matter what timeless work of art or architecture is in view. Mid-afternoon arrives, the heart of the night according to the traveler's brain, and a nap seems the ticket. A comforting seven or eight hours later the traveler awakes, refreshed, to a city in darkness. Where can breakfast be found at midnight?

The discrepancy between the cycle of sleep and wakefulness controlled by the brain and "clock time" is known as jet lag. When at home, biological clocks and wristwatches work in harmony, but once in a new time zone the two desynchronize. With body rhythms out of tune, the traveler has a hard time battling the strong influences of human physiology.

Body temperature falls at bedtime, as does metabolic rate. Hormones, blood count and heartbeat, along with physical dexterity and mental alertness, all follow a circadian, or daily, pattern set by the brain. These physiological functions control the desire to sleep or wake according to a biological clock; desynchronization leaves the traveler feeling dull, tired and irritable.

The internal time-keeping device depends on certain brain activities which have not been precisely pinned down, but the effects of the biological clock are evident. What is commonly known as jet lag today has long been experienced by factory workers who alternated from day to night shifts. Desynchronization among factory workers is very similar to that of the overseas traveler—both experience a shift in sleep schedules. Workers face mood swings, problems with alertness, lack of creativity, and in severe cases, ulcers, depression, anxiety and sleep disorders.

Gaining full rhythm synchronization is important for jet-setters, as well as for those who have no choice but to alternate work schedules. On average, one full day of recovery should be allotted for each hour of the time shift. For travelers on a short visit or workers who shift frequently resynchronization may be a problem.

Keeping in sync with the world is easier for some than for others. Younger people have an easier time handling effects of jet lag than older people because their bio-rhythms adjust more rapidly. People with a high tolerance for shifting schedules have a greater range of body temperature. Analysis of time-shifts show that resynchronization is faster for westbound flights. The reason is that the suprachiasmatic nuclei—a pair of neuron clusters occupying the space of a pinhead in the hypothalamus—find it easier to "phase-delay", or turn back the clock, than to "phase-advance." Timed exposure of the suprachiasmatic nuclei to bright lights has been shown to reset the circadian rhythms by as much as 12 hours in 3 days.

Not enough is known about biological clocks to be able to reset them regularly and reliably, but with research lighting the path, the flexible brain may well keep up with the supersonic age.

as a restorative. This secretion likely takes place during the delta stage of non-REM sleep. A person whose slow-wave Stage 3 sleep is repeatedly curtailed or interrupted over weeks or months begins to experience overall muscular aches.

A whole class of physical and mental disorders is related to sleep. Some, like insomnia and sleep apnea, are relatively common. Sleep apnea can occur at any age, but the majority of cases develop in males after age 40 and consist of periodic halts in breathing that may last for 15 to 120 seconds. These episodes may occur hundreds of times a night without the sleeper's being aware, and may result from a failure in the respiratory centers of the brain or, perhaps, excessive relaxation

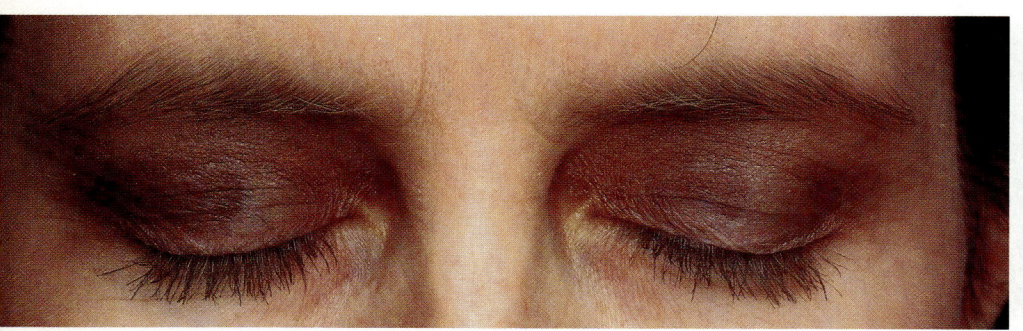
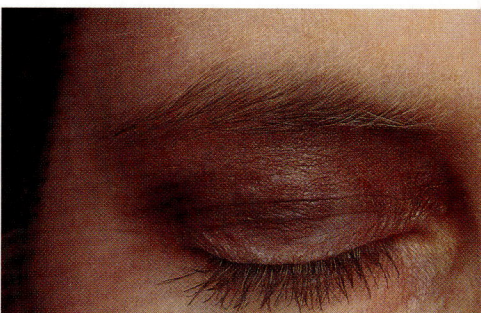

Scientists remain baffled by the rapid eye movement that occurs during the dream stage. All birds and mammals experience REM sleep, often accompanied by dreams. Cold-blooded animals have no dreams; sharks do not even sleep.

of muscles in the throat, which consequently collapses on itself and blocks the passage of air. Other sleep disorders, including narcolepsy—episodes of uncontrollable sleep that strike at inappropriate times—are far more rare.

Even some complex psychological disorders such as depression have strong connections with disordered sleep. Major symptoms of depression are insomnia and early morning waking. Brain-wave monitoring reveals that depressed people display abnormal timing of REM and delta sleep that often commences just a few minutes after they enter their first round of non-REM sleep. Support for the hypothesis that out-of-kilter REM and non-REM cycles could cause depression comes from several experiments in which researchers temporarily relieved depression by either depriving patients of sleep or forcing them to stay awake an hour later each night. There is also the likelihood that the sleep and mood systems of the brain share a common neurochemistry that, when out of balance, produces both a depressed mood and poor sleep.

As the brain ages, its need for sleep of all types falls off somewhat. While newborn human infants spend more than 50 percent of their 16 to 18 hours' sleep per day in REM sleep, adults spend only one and a half to two hours in REM. In old age, the REM percentage stays constant (although the total amount of sleep may fall below six hours). Slow-wave non-REM sleep may disappear altogether. The elderly report waking frequently during the night and often complain that they do not get enough sleep. Ironically, sleeping pills, which are supposed to address this problem, only make things worse. Neurochemists have found that barbiturates in particular suppress REM sleep and eliminate the most restful stages of non-REM. Newer hypnotic drugs, such as the benzodiazepenes—including Valium—partially correct this failing, but the search is on for other substances that will induce sleep without deranging its essential rhythms.

One of the strangest sleep disorders is somnambulism, or sleepwalking, when the sleeper rises from bed and moves about heedless of others, expressionless but with eyes wide open, sometimes performing complex tasks like housecleaning without being aware. It was long thought that sleepwalkers were acting out dreams, but sleep clinicians have discovered that somnambulism occurs during the deepest stages of non-REM sleep, classically beginning when brain waves settle into the slow rhythm of delta sleep. Although it is not yet known what causes the sleeping brain to send out the barrage of motor impulses that might cause someone to rise from bed and tour the house, researchers have dispelled the old wives' tale that sleepwalkers should not be disturbed lest they suffer a fatal shock. Although hard

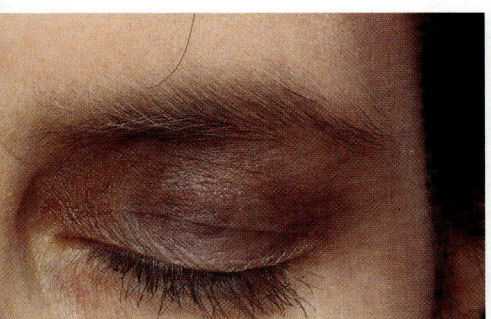
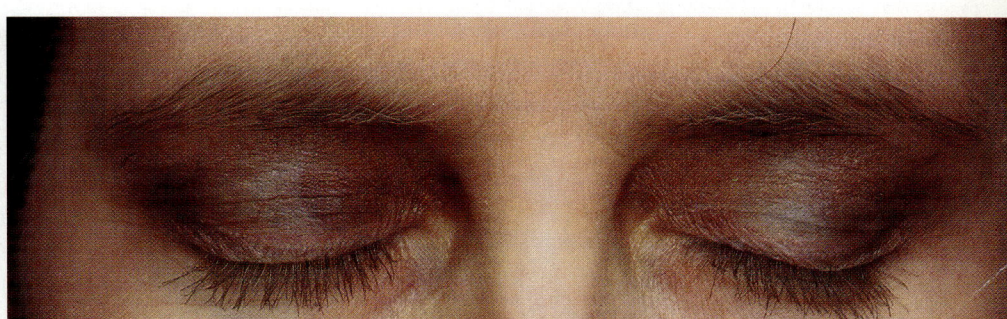

to rouse, sleepwalkers can be wakened safely. In the morning, though, they may recall little about their nocturnal rambles.

In a newly identified sleep disorder, REM behavior disorder, people actually act out their dreams. The normal muscle paralysis of REM sleep is lost, enabling the sleeper to carry out what is being dreamed—often leading to injury.

THE STUFF OF DREAMS

When Kleitman and Aserinsky discovered REM sleep, they also discovered the source of those varied and elusive phantasms whose meaning has been debated for millennia: dreams. In so doing, they dispelled the myths and conjectures that had accumulated over thousands of years as people sought to explain their nightly slide into a state sometimes closer to insanity than rationality.

More than a diverting light show, dreaming is a process that engages almost the entire brain. It is a veritable firestorm of electrochemical activity, originating from deep within the brain, which sweeps over the higher, cortical regions. Neurons barrage one another with signals at a pace often outstripping their daytime mark. So vigorous are these exertions that some researchers have deemed dreaming "the third state of existence."

On an electroencephalogram, the onset of dreams is signaled by the sudden shift from the slower waves of non-REM to the faster waves of REM. These sharp, closely spaced waves markedly resemble those produced by the awake brain. Clusters of neurons in the pons section of the brainstem bombard the higher brain with messages. In response, the specialized centers in the cortex run at full pitch, striving to keep up with the incoming information. They send out signals to trigger walking and running motions in the muscles, but at the same time the brainstem sends out signals that prevent the muscles from moving. They also activate various bodily systems, such as that responsible for respiration.

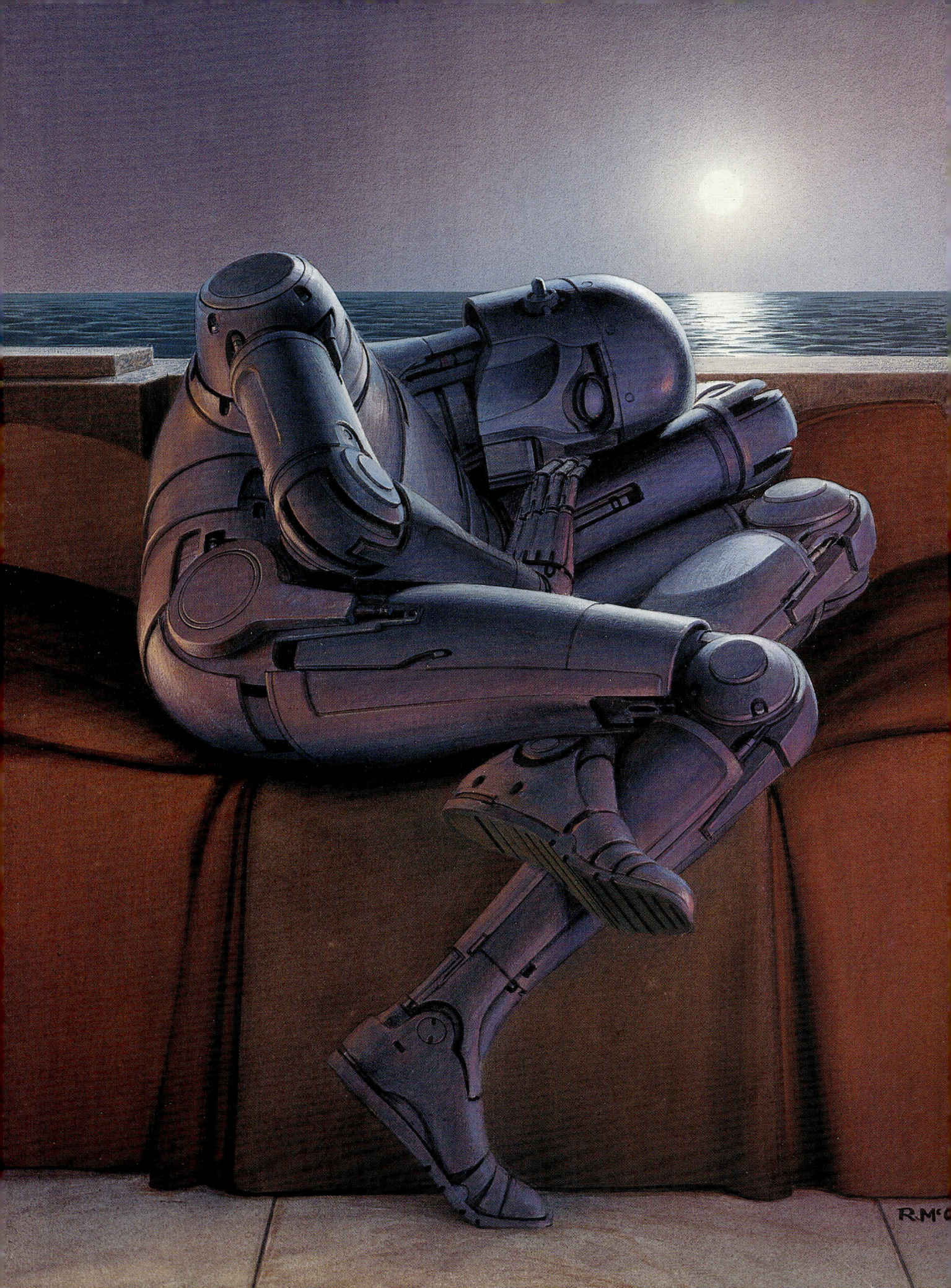

Too Little...

Americans request 24 million prescriptions for sleeping pills every year. Though everyone experiences some sleeplessness when stress or excitement overstimulates the arousal system, some unfortunate individuals suffer chronic insomnia. The problem may be due to behavioral disturbances, or a variety of medical disorders, including mental depression.

In the desperate search for magical sleep potions, insomniacs have discovered warm milk, chamomile tea and counting sheep. But experts do not recommend alcohol as a sleep inducer because it results in a fragmented, less restful sleep. In fact, virtually all classes of drugs that promote sleep also have the potential to disturb sleep patterns.

The ultimate sleeping pill, a natural sleep-inducing chemical, actually may exist in the body. Some biochemists think this agent (still unidentified) accumulates in the body during the day and finally puts us to sleep at night.

Now there appears to be dark at the end of the tunnel for those who toss and turn their way to sleep. Scientists speculate that for some insomniacs the biological clock, which regulates the sleep-wake cycle, may be out of kilter. In one study, insomniacs passed through the wake-maintenance zone—a period, usually in the evening, during which sleep is difficult—about 3.6 hours later than normal. Researchers have found that sitting

...Too Much

under bright lights (48 times the intensity of normal room light) helps to reset the sleeper's biological clock.

While many insomniacs have trouble sleeping for days on end, a few suffer from total insomnia, claiming to have gone without definable sleep for many years. Jesus de Frutos, a Spaniard afflicted with this condition, says he has only dozed since 1954.

At the other end of the sleep scale, a narcoleptic plods wearily through another day, feeling sluggish regardless of the number of hours he slept the previous night. And when the urge to doze becomes overwhelming, the narcoleptic succumbs to sleep, disrupting whatever he is doing.

Crippled by excessive daytime sleepiness, narcoleptics are often prevented from performing the most normal activities, such as driving a car or holding a job. Other disabling symptoms of this condition include cataplexy (temporary paralysis triggered by emotional arousal), sleep paralysis and frightening hallucinations at the beginning or the end of a sleep period.

Recent neurochemical findings suggest that two mechanisms underlie narcolepsy. In a study of narcoleptic dogs, daytime sleepiness seemed to be related to an abnormality in the release of dopamine, the chemical messenger associated with alertness.

Dreaming, and the muscle paralysis which accompanies it, normally occur during REM sleep. In narcolepsy, these phenomena are triggered while the person is still awake. Paralysis sets in before sleep onset or following waking, and dreaming is experienced as hallucinating. Preliminary trials with a drug which increases dopamine activity while inhibiting acetylcholine turnover have shown promising results.

Although not considered a symptom of narcolepsy, sleep apnea is experienced more frequently by narcoleptics than other members of the general population. This condition, characterized by intermittent cessation of breathing during sleep—sometimes up to 190 seconds at a time, as many as 600 times a night—robs the sleeper of much-needed rest. In severe cases, certain abnormal physical conditions associated with sleep apnea—low blood-oxygen content, hypertension, slow heartbeat—are suspected as a possible cause of death.

SLEEPYHEAD
Sleep, at times elusive, at times overwhelming, is a natural biological phenomenon. Problem sleepers are the subject of new research.

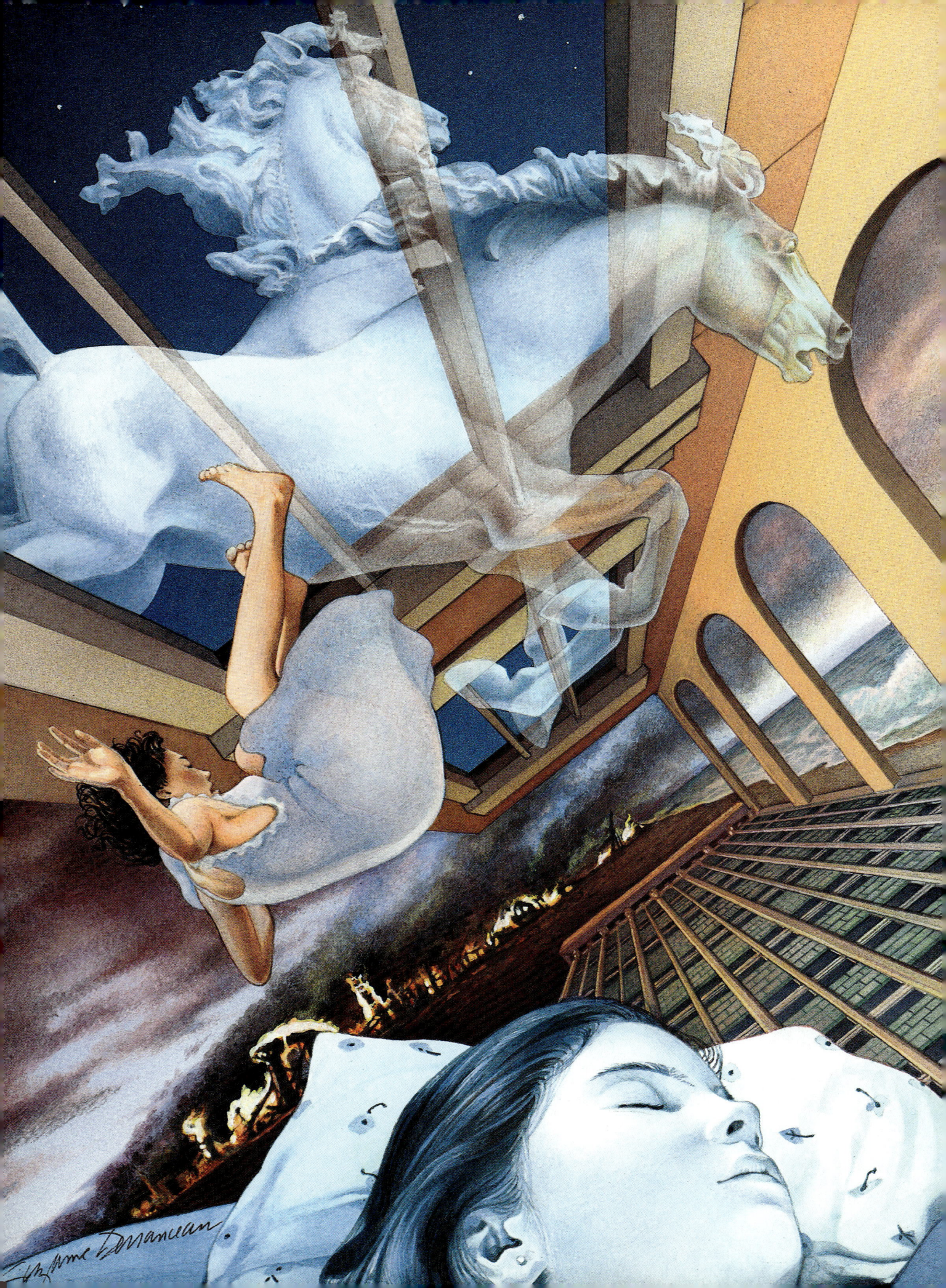

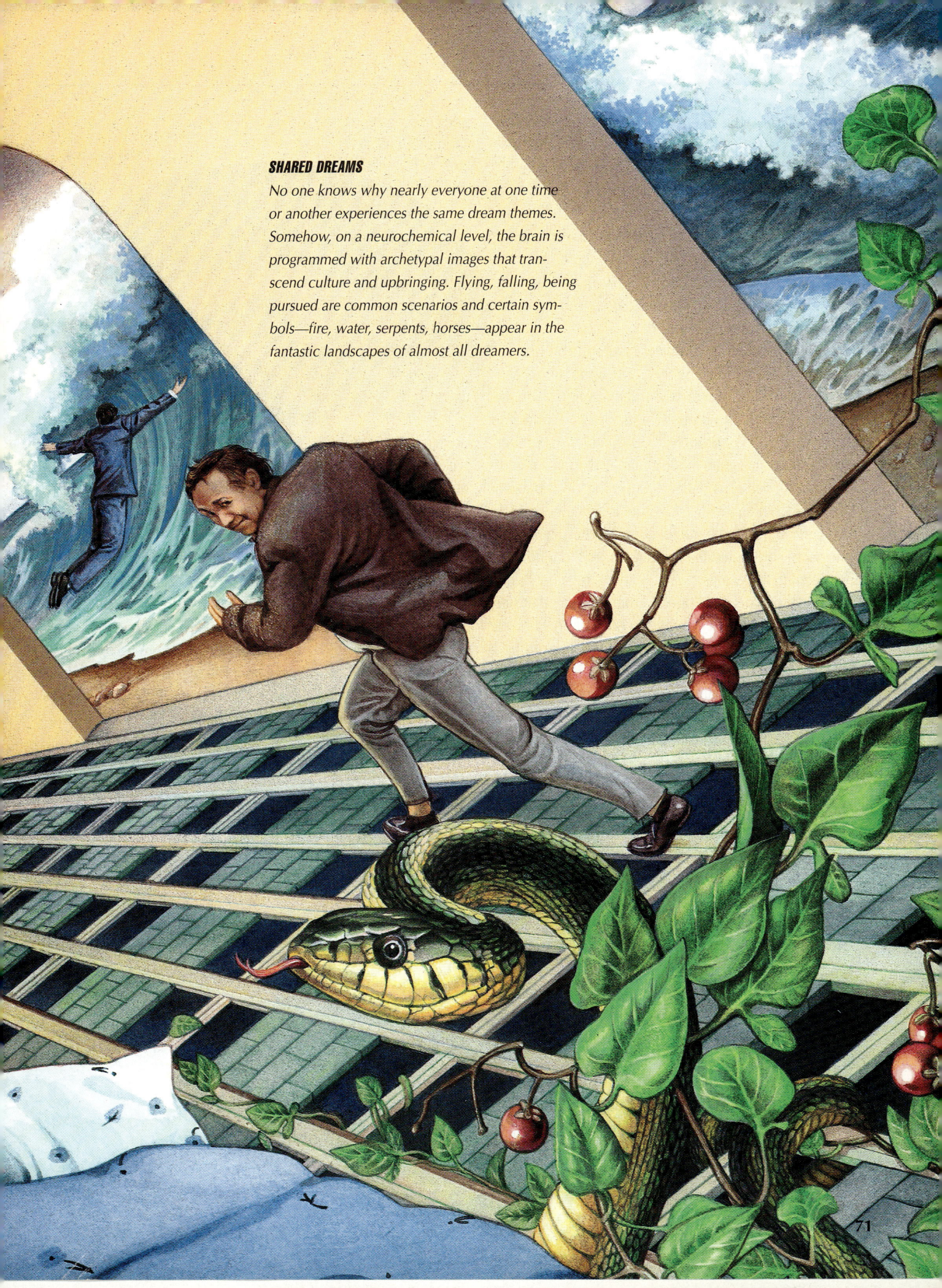

SHARED DREAMS

No one knows why nearly everyone at one time or another experiences the same dream themes. Somehow, on a neurochemical level, the brain is programmed with archetypal images that transcend culture and upbringing. Flying, falling, being pursued are common scenarios and certain symbols—fire, water, serpents, horses—appear in the fantastic landscapes of almost all dreamers.

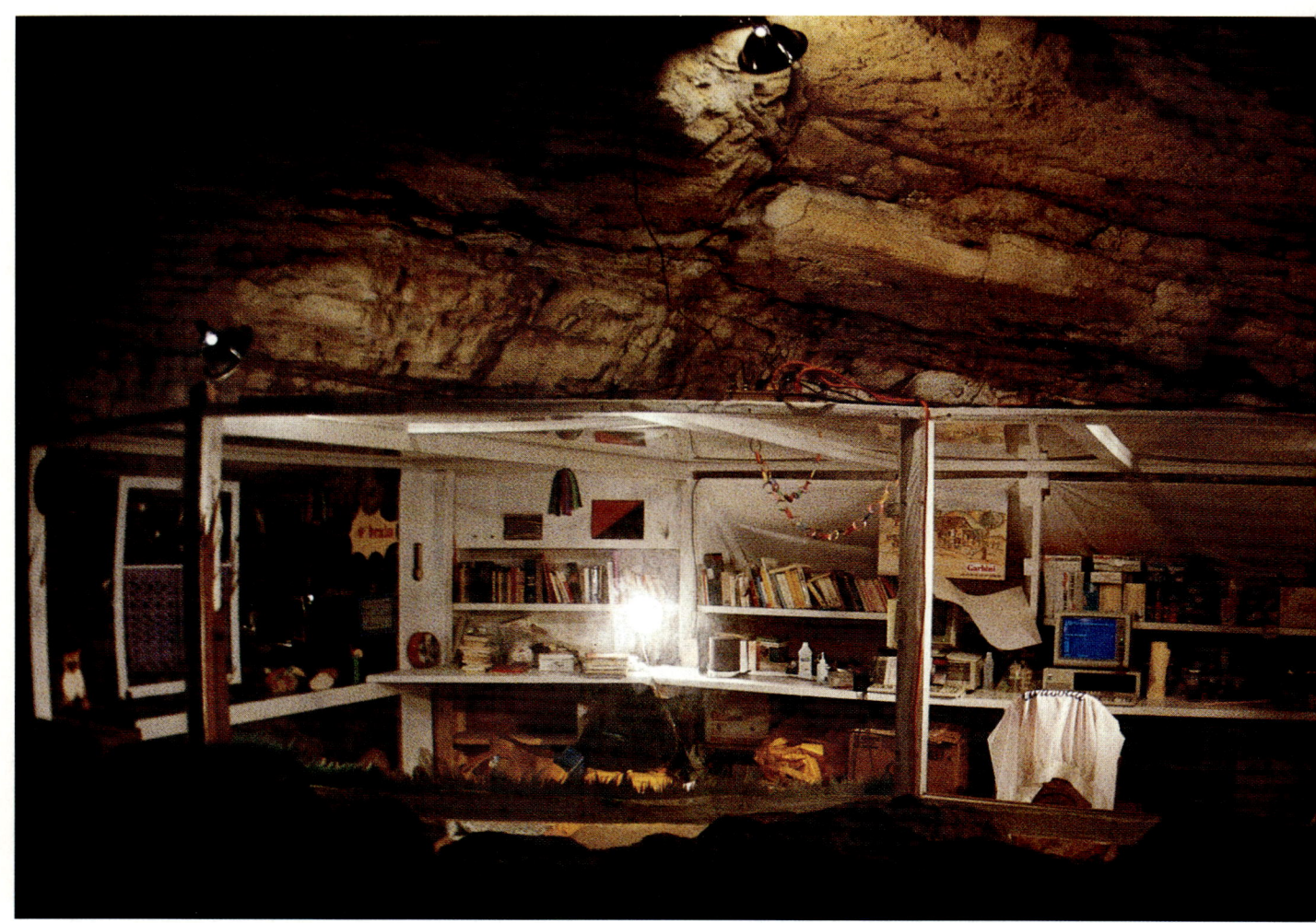

¿Siesta? ¡Sí!

Scientists who study the brain's internal clock are giving business a wake-up call. Once common in many cultures, the siesta is dying at the hand of industrialization. Yet by pushing for uniform, unbroken work periods, corporations and governments may be cutting productivity, rather than boosting it. Sleep researchers now say napping is a natural tonic for body and soul—and potentially good for profits.

Evidence supporting afternoon sleep arose from studies following the cycles of sleepiness and wakefulness throughout each day. Deprived of clocks, natural light and other time cues, volunteers in subterranean clinics follow their own biological rhythms. Over the course of a few weeks, sleep naturally breaks into two daily sessions—a long block during the night and a much shorter period of one or two hours in the afternoon. On average, the onset of the afternoon nap-attack occurs 12 hours after the middle of the night sleep. So, for a person who sleeps from midnight until seven a.m., the urge to doze off strikes at three to four p.m. Afternoon sleep is usually dreamless, deep and restful, characterized by the slow, regular delta waves of Stage 4 sleep. The only known drawback to afternoon napping is "sleep inertia," a temporary stupor that may occur on awakening. Grogginess and disorientation may last up to 15 minutes.

Once the drugged sensation has lifted, the brain functions at peak performance. Energy, alertness, sustained attention span, greater decisiveness and cheerfulness are among the post-nap rewards cited by researchers, who predict that industry itself, by ignoring such benefits, has been asleep at the switch.

STATES OF MIND

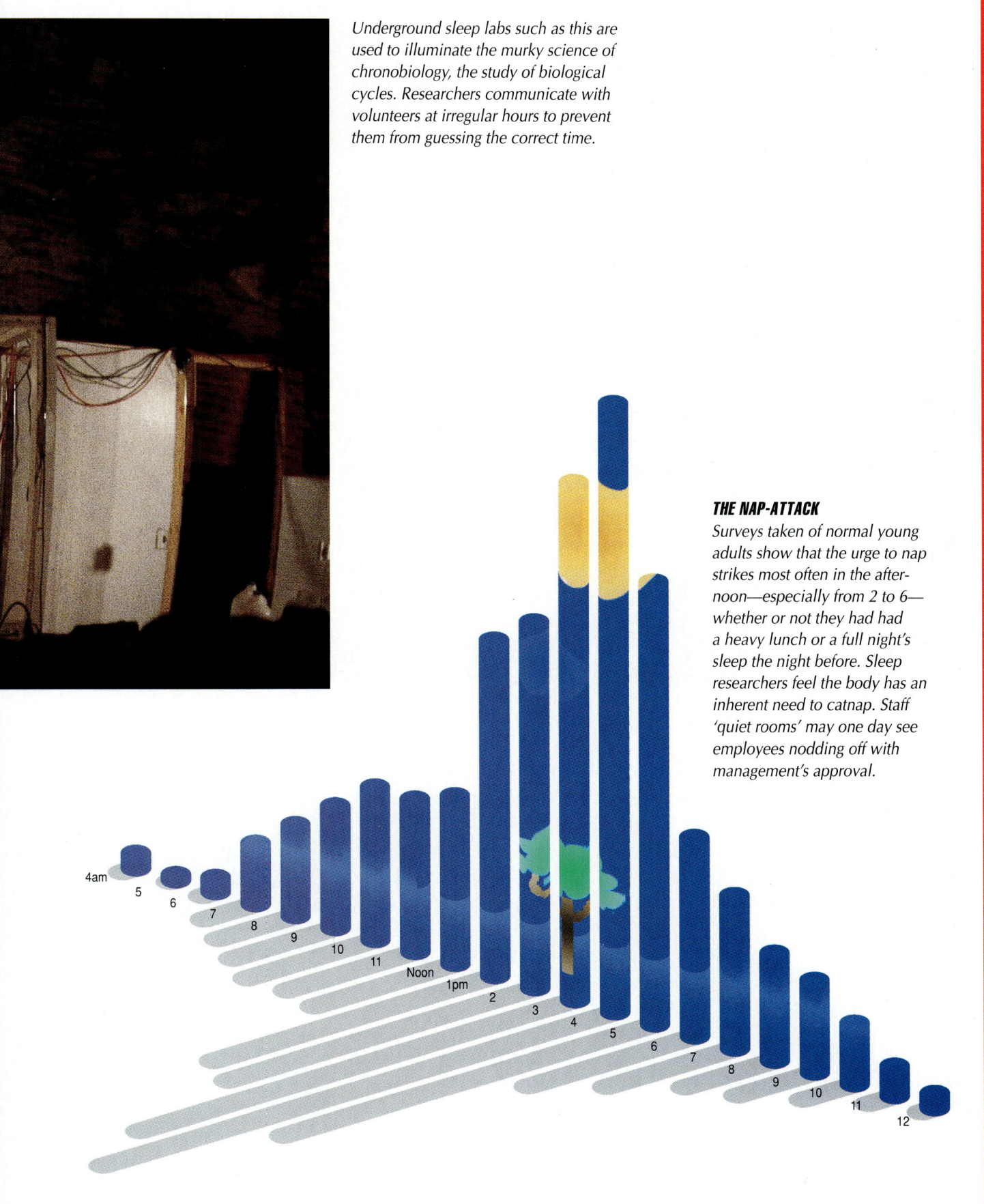

Underground sleep labs such as this are used to illuminate the murky science of chronobiology, the study of biological cycles. Researchers communicate with volunteers at irregular hours to prevent them from guessing the correct time.

THE NAP-ATTACK
Surveys taken of normal young adults show that the urge to nap strikes most often in the afternoon—especially from 2 to 6—whether or not they had had a heavy lunch or a full night's sleep the night before. Sleep researchers feel the body has an inherent need to catnap. Staff 'quiet rooms' may one day see employees nodding off with management's approval.

MOOD, MOLECULES AND MADNESS

Shortly before noon on a blazing August day in 1966, a muscular, blond, engineering student named Charles Whitman ascended the 30-story observation tower at the University of Texas in Austin. Beside him on the elevator were his old Marine Corps duffel bag and foot locker, both loaded with provisions and weaponry: a bowie knife, a machete, three pistols, three high-powered rifles, a sawed-off shotgun and 700 rounds of ammunition. At the entrance to the observation deck he took out a rifle and used it to bludgeon a receptionist to death. Then he lugged his arsenal onto the deck. Positioning himself at the south parapet, he opened fire, blasting students and sightseers on the campus below for the next hour and a half.

Before he was stopped by a barrage of police bullets, Whitman had killed 12 people and wounded 33. The previous evening he had executed his mother and knifed his young wife to death. It was a horrifying episode of mass murder.

What happened? What circuits in Whitman's 25-year-old brain misfired to engender this lethal convulsion of rage and aggression? There was little in his background to explain it. He had been a model youth, though known for his short temper. But nothing in his past seemed to account for the blood-spattered pathways around the university tower.

Yet, in one of the ironies of emotional disturbance, Whitman himself had sensed what was coming. That spring he had visited a university psychiatrist, seeking to curb his aggressive moods. Then, on the eve of his rampage, he sat down at his typewriter. "I've been having fears and violent impulses," he wrote. "I've had some tremendous headaches. I am prepared to die. After my death I wish an autopsy to be performed to see if there's any mental disorder."

Though armchair explainers tended to look for psychiatric causes, it was Whitman's autopsy that was profoundly revealing. Deep within his brain, in the region of his hypothalamus, was a tumor the size of a walnut. The hypothalamus, as research now shows, is a vital link in the complex circuitry that regulates emotion.

The human face—even a very young one—can be a barometer of emotion or an elusive veil. Though scientists do not have a complete picture of how feelings work, they do know that every conscious thought carries some emotional tag.

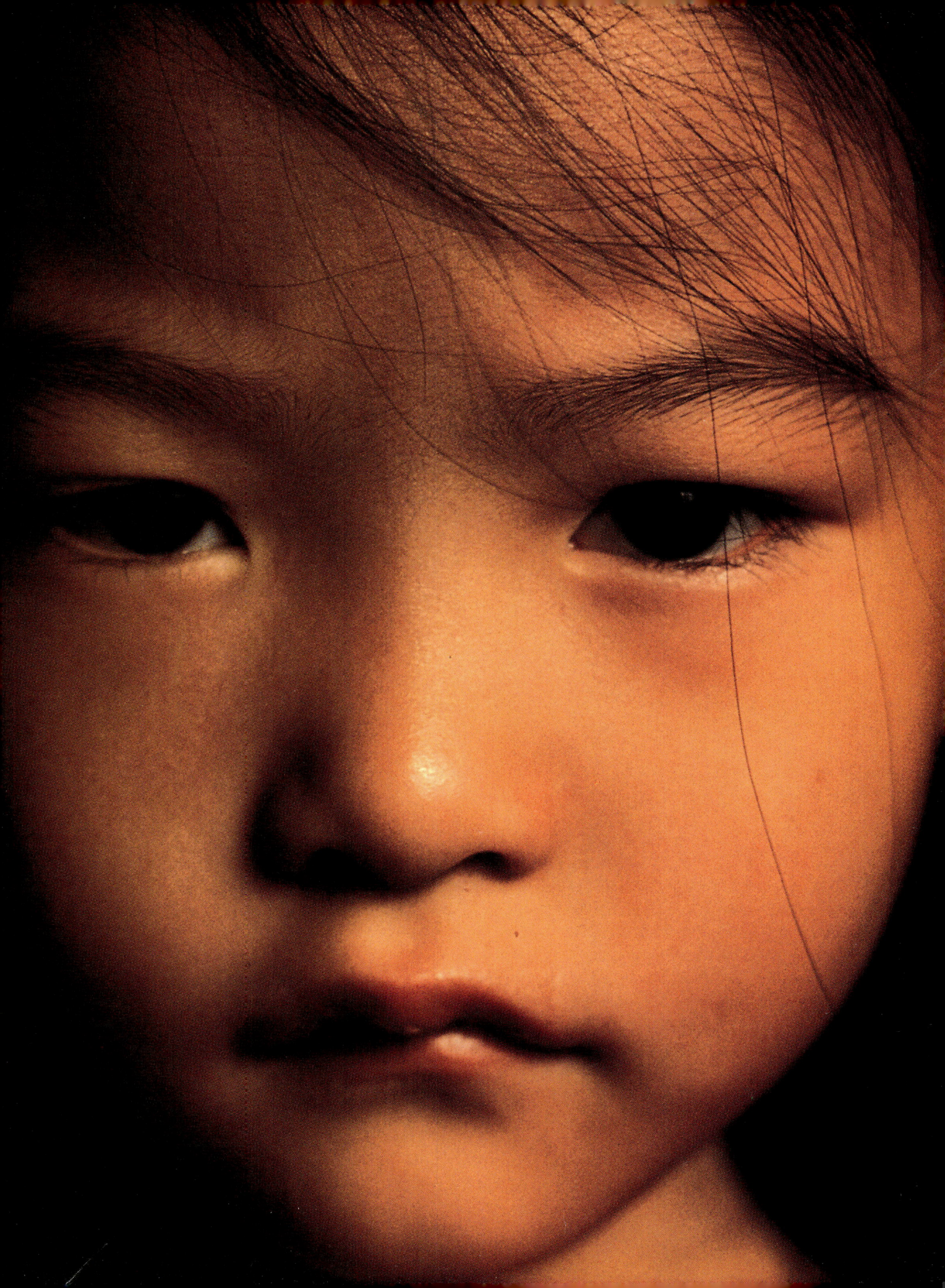

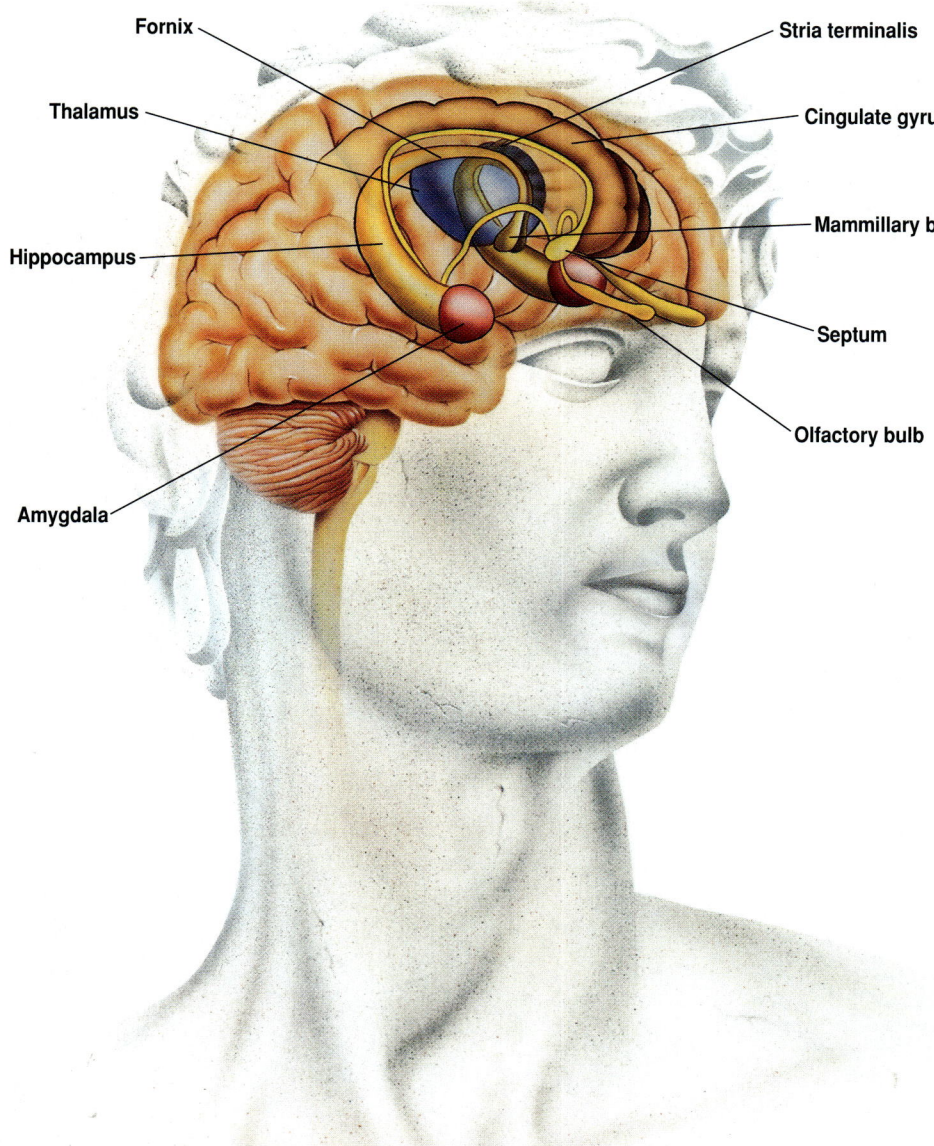

THE LIMBIC SYSTEM
Neurotransmission affecting mood occurs principally in a circuit of structures known collectively as the limbic system. Experiments using electrodes have pinpointed the septum as a key pleasure center.

Stimulation of an electrode inserted into this structure can send a test animal—or a human volunteer—into paroxysms of fear and anger.

No one has yet come up with a complete picture of how emotions operate, nor even a scientifically precise definition of just what emotion is. Yet its effects are all-pervasive. Every thought that filters through the mind, every sensation that penetrates the consciousness, takes on some degree of emotional coloring. Feelings are what give value to life, separating the important from the inconsequential. All behavior derives from them. "Our entire psychical activity is bent upon procuring pleasure and avoiding pain," wrote Sigmund Freud a century ago, and his observation holds true for every human endeavor. Even the most tedious chores of daily existence—commuting to work, cramming for an exam—are undertaken in hope of future satisfaction.

Most of the time—in a healthy mind—a balance prevails between the forces of emotion and the realities of life. Information from the senses travels through synapses, picks up a cargo of feeling, rendezvous with the centers of memory, and motivates responses that are sensible and benign. But on occasion the feelings can be overwhelming and self-defeating. A severe psychic reversal, from the loss of a job to the death of a loved one, can plunge its victim into an immobilizing state of darkest melancholy.

Most recover as, with time, the brain's circuits regain their equilibrium. But in some people the feelings run riot, taking full and permanent control. The black mood may deepen and become habitual. Or it may swing into a frenetic euphoria. The stresses of life may wear down the psyche and erode the health, bringing on ulcers or heart attack. Some people, in their search for pleasure, may turn to the swift chemical thrills of narcotics, only to find themselves embarked on the downward spiral of addiction. And on occasion the mind may snap, drifting off into a world of fantasy and numb, internal terror. Or it may explode with the murderous violence of a Charles Whitman.

FEELINGS

The poet Emily Dickinson knew the highs and lows of intense emotion. A spinster in a 19th-Century New England town, and given to bouts of depression, she recorded her fears and perceptions in brief, tightly worded verses of remarkable power. For her, emotion was a physical experience: "If I read a book and it makes my whole body so cold no fire can ever warm me, I know it is poetry. If I feel physically as if the top of my head were taken off, I know this is poetry."

The idea that feelings have a physical basis goes back to ancient times. Hippocrates believed that mood was controlled by four bodily fluids, which he called humors. An ample supply of blood made a person sanguine: ruddy-complexioned, brave, optimistic, amorous. An excess of mucus, or phlegm, tended to make him cold, sluggish and dull—in a word, phlegmatic. If a person was sad, he suffered from excess black bile. Yellow bile caused him to be quick-tempered and choleric. So convincing was this scheme that it lasted into the 17th Century.

Besides his theory of humors, Hippocrates proposed an even more significant idea—that the brain is the organ of thought and feeling. This was a bold assertion at the time since no less an authority than Aristotle had decided that thoughts and feelings resided in the heart. The question persisted. "Tell me where is fancy bred," asked Shakespeare in the *Merchant of Venice*, "in the heart or in the head?"

Even today the division is not clear-cut, so closely are the body and the mind interconnected. Back in the 1800s the American psychologist William James awarded first place to the mind. But he viewed the initial emotion as a purely physical response, which the mind then interpreted. "We feel sorry because we cry," James said, "angry because we strike, afraid because we tremble."

Further research showed the process to be considerably more complicated. In 1929 the physiologist Walter Cannon pointed out that the same physical response may accompany a multitude of different emotions. A Beethoven sonata may cause the scalp to tingle, but so can watching a horror film. Cannon decided that the initial nerve impulses travel first to the thalamus, then considered to be the brain's main switchboard. There they split, he suggested, with some going to the cerebral cortex, the seat of cognition, and others heading for the hypothalamus, the producer of physiological changes.

But that is only half the story. If the hypothalamus is key to emotional response, so are a dozen or more brain structures that surround it. The neurologist who first explored the connections between them was James W. Papez of Chicago. Writing in the late 1930s, Papez noted that patients with damage in this section of the brain were prone to sudden emotional outbursts. One formation that caught his attention was the hippocampus, the S-shaped body—vaguely resembling a seahorse—that circles the thalamus. He also focused on an adjacent area of the cortex known as the cingulate gyrus. Both are closely connected to the thalamus, the hypothalamus, and certain key areas of the midbrain and brainstem. Emotion, Papez decided, is a stream of nerve impulses running through these various circuits.

It was a brilliant hypothesis, and it forms the basis for today's neurological picture of emotional response. Other structures have been added to the original Papez circuit: the almond-shaped amygdala, significant in feelings of both fear and aggression; the septum, which may hold the key to pleasure and pain; other areas of the cortex; and numerous sites in the brainstem. Together they make up the limbic system—so called because it lies at the limbus, or threshold, between the forebrain and the more primitive regions beneath.

According to the current scheme, emotions arise in the limbic circuits, in response to various neural stimuli. Neural pathways lead from there to the frontal lobes of the cortex, which monitor the feelings, shape them and interpret them. These two brain areas then exert their influence on the hypothalamus, which in turn transmits the messages that trigger appropriate physical responses.

The pioneering genius on the limbic system is Paul MacLean, of the Laboratory of Clinical Science in Maryland. The human brain, MacLean reasons, is a product of long development that began with the most primitive life forms. The reptilian brain, largely restricted to the brainstem, is the site of the instincts. Feeding and fighting, the instinctive rituals of courtship and aggression, the urge to dominate and the postures of submission—all these come under its sway. Such behavior is unconscious and automatic, "wired in" through the brainstem's circuits. It includes everything from a lizard's compulsion to puff out its neck scruff when it meets another lizard, to the macho preening of a streetwise male teenager.

Reptiles have no feelings in MacLean's scheme, but most or all mammals probably do. And while the reptilian brain is locked into involuntary, programmed responses, the limbic brain enjoys the benefits of flexibility and intent. "One of the peculiar characteristics of the emotions," MacLean observes, "is that they are not neutral. Emotions are either agreeable or disagreeable." The limbic system thus serves as a judge, monitoring the quality of each sensory event. All mammals, including humans, take their cue from its signals, and modify their behavior in order to promote well-being.

Evidence of the limbic system's role in the search for emotional satisfaction came to light by chance, in one of the great serendipitous discoveries of neurology. In 1953 Dr. James Olds, a researcher at McGill University in Montreal, was studying the role of the brain in learning. In an experiment on a rat, he implanted an electrode into what he thought was its hypothalamus and applied current. Under normal circumstances, the rat should have shied away in alarm. Instead, it sought the stimulus again and again.

A postmortem revealed the reason. By chance the electrode had ended up in the front portion of the hypothalamus, just where it connects to another limbic structure called the septum. What was even stranger was that electrical stimulation of the hypothalamus in previous tests had usually sent the animal into a snarling, spitting, teeth-chattering rage. Could the septum be the brain's pleasure center, a kind of command post that mediates the quest for emotional well-being?

To test this idea, Olds put another rat—with a similarly implanted electrode—in a cage with a large lever that allowed the rat to turn on the electricity itself. The rat pushed the lever incessantly, as many as a hundred times a minute, for hours on end, until it was exhausted. Nor were rats the only animals to behave this way. Rabbits, dogs, dolphins, monkeys, even human patient volunteers, often feel intense elation whenever they turn on the current.

Though the septum appeared to be connected to pleasure, other areas of the limbic brain seemed to harbor more negative feelings. As far back as 1928, researchers discovered that a small electric charge delivered into certain sections of a cat's hypothalamus will cause the animal to arch its back, lash its tail and launch a frenzied attack on the nearest living creature. Pain seems to register largely in the thalamus. Stimulation in other areas has been shown to prompt feelings of anguish, foreboding, loneliness, apathy and despair.

One seemingly all-purpose trigger is the amygdala. Like the septum, the amygdala contains a high concentration of pleasure-mediating neurons. At the same time, it is associated with displays of both anger and fear. A laboratory monkey, when electrically stimulated in this region, may cringe, grunt, twitch, growl, gag, hiss or urinate, depending on the strength of the current and the exact spot where it is applied. Surgical removal of the amygdala, on the other hand, may utterly transform a normally aggressive animal, making it gentle and affectionate.

Outside the laboratory, nature provides its own examples of wayward electrical stimulation. The most dramatic, perhaps, is epilepsy, a chaotic firing of neurons that has been likened to a lightning storm in the brain. The seizures may be mild or severe, but in most cases the victim remains passive. On occasion, however, the problem can be devastating, as was the case with a particular 21-year-old epileptic patient named Julie.

The daughter of a physician, Julie was subject to attacks that would send her into a blind, paranoid frenzy. In one, she stabbed a bystander with a dinner knife—then woke up dazed, not knowing what she had done. During her treatment, neurologists found that the epileptic discharges were coming from the area of her amygdala. An electrode probe isolated the spot; when the electricity was turned on Julie would first grow quietly hostile. Then, as the seizure took hold, she would smash things or pound the wall with her fists. A simple surgical procedure using heat and radio frequency current destroyed the abnormal tissue and cured Julie of both her violence and her severe epilepsy.

In the light of such examples, it seems only natural to think of the brain's emotional apparatus as a series of independent neurological centers—pleasure spots and pain sites, anger areas and fear nodes. But this is not the whole picture. One problem is duplication; too many sites appear to control the same emotion, while

THE UPS . . .

The heights of euphoria are experienced by nearly everyone at some point. Only when a person's mood escalates into a protracted, uncontrollable high does it constitute a problem.

any one site may trigger a broad spectrum of emotional responses. Emotions cannot be localized in individual bits of brain matter. Instead, they emanate from a number of different areas working in concert—or, more precisely, from the neural pathways that crisscross the limbic system and lead out from it.

The controlling factor in the flow of information within the brain is the same set of substances that carries signals throughout the nervous system—chemical neurotransmitters. They are the modern version of Hippocrates' four humors, except that their number is far greater than Hippocrates ever imagined. Though about 40 neurotransmitters have already been identified, most probably there are several hundred more waiting to be uncovered by researchers. Some activate the nerve cells, causing them to fire, some shut the signals off. By activating or shutting down the firing, they act as chemical intermediaries. Some also facilitate the effect of others. Working together, they orchestrate the shifting moods and attitudes that accompany daily existence.

Chemicals of various types have been influencing people's moods ever since their tribal ancestors began sparking up the evenings with mead or fermented grape juice. But the way chemicals work has been a discovery of the last several decades. It has come, in large part, as a byproduct of a pressing situation—the need for drugs that can relieve the agonizing symptoms of mental illness.

A surprising variety of mental disorders seem to have a chemical basis. Back in the early 1900s, fully 10 percent of psychiatric inmates in the American South suffered from pellagra, a condition marked by hallucinations, delirium and rapid swings of mood. Most of the pellagra patients came from poor backgrounds where diets were skimpy; in particular, they lacked the B vitamin niacin, essential for proper nerve function. When this was discovered, the cure became obvious. Given supplements of niacin, the patients recovered.

Mood disorders include a broad spectrum of ailments, and pellagra is just one of them. The most prevalent today is depression, an apathy and gloom of clinical proportions. By some estimates, as many as one out of four people may suffer from it at some point in their lives. In severe cases the black moods reach suicidal intensity; 16 percent of depression victims, if untreated, eventually kill themselves. In another 10 percent, the gloom will alternate with periods of manic euphoria, which themselves can be almost as destructive. Here thoughts and emotions race through the brain "like shooting stars," as one manic patient put it, until they spin out of control. Feelings of confidence, power, energy, generosity, cleverness and general superiority sweep beyond the bounds of rational fact—until suddenly everything collapses, leaving the victim in psychic shambles.

Everyone experiences moments of elation or discouragement, in most cases attributable to some external event. A success at the office brings a sense of well-being; any important loss creates sadness. But victims of true mania or depression are more vulnerable to minor and major stresses; occasionally there is no discernible outside cause, and this in itself contributes to the feeling of hopelessness. The swings in mood are generated internally, by the brain itself.

The thought that moods may be chemically induced gained prominence in the late 1940s, after a chance discovery in Melbourne, Australia. Dr. John Cade, a physician at a psychiatric ward there, was conducting an experiment to see whether some toxic agent in the blood of his manic patients was causing their

. . . AND DOWNS
A moderate ebb and flow of mood is as natural as the tides, but excessive worry can aggravate a minor low into a full-blown funk. Chemical imbalance is often an underlying cause.

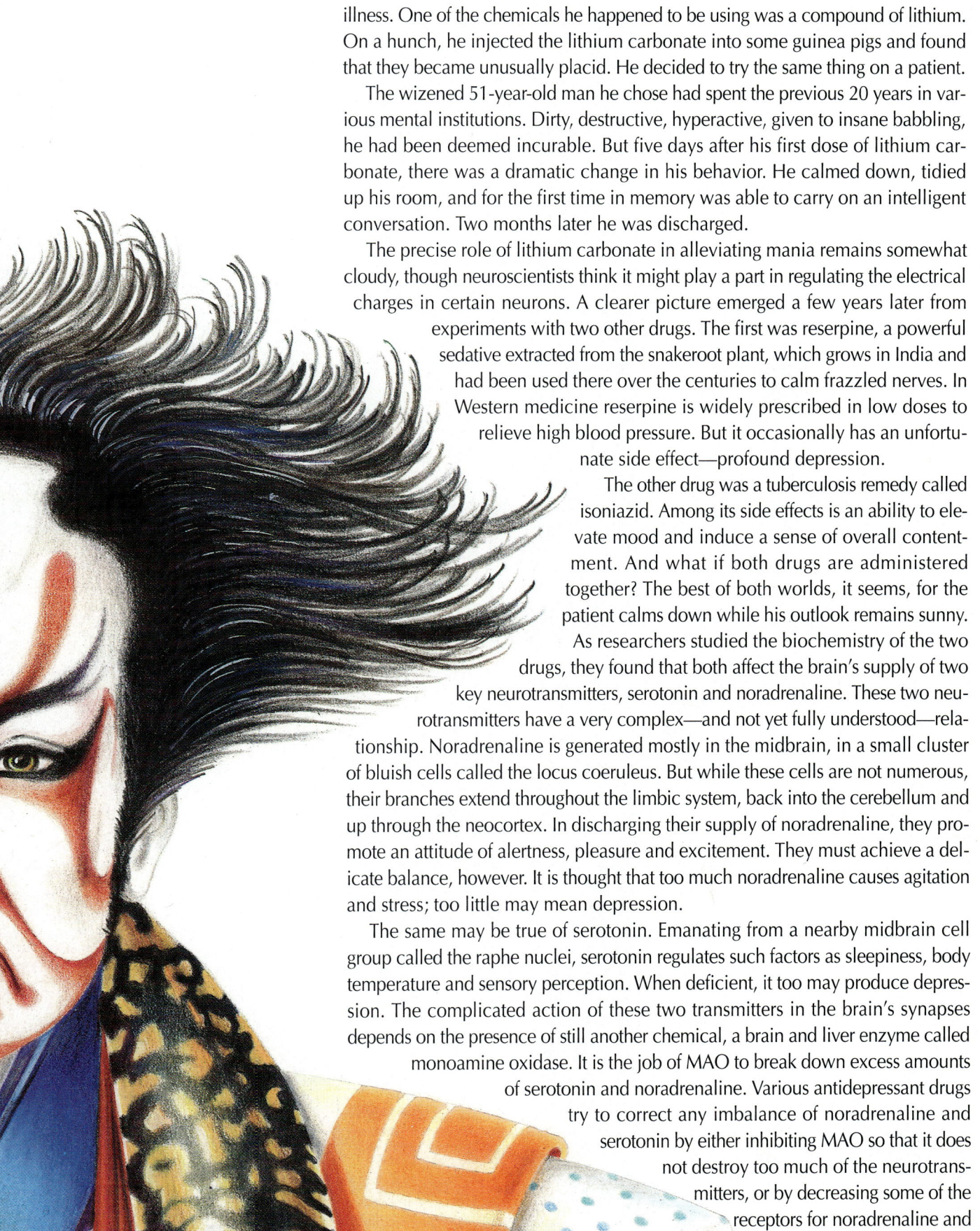

illness. One of the chemicals he happened to be using was a compound of lithium. On a hunch, he injected the lithium carbonate into some guinea pigs and found that they became unusually placid. He decided to try the same thing on a patient.

The wizened 51-year-old man he chose had spent the previous 20 years in various mental institutions. Dirty, destructive, hyperactive, given to insane babbling, he had been deemed incurable. But five days after his first dose of lithium carbonate, there was a dramatic change in his behavior. He calmed down, tidied up his room, and for the first time in memory was able to carry on an intelligent conversation. Two months later he was discharged.

The precise role of lithium carbonate in alleviating mania remains somewhat cloudy, though neuroscientists think it might play a part in regulating the electrical charges in certain neurons. A clearer picture emerged a few years later from experiments with two other drugs. The first was reserpine, a powerful sedative extracted from the snakeroot plant, which grows in India and had been used there over the centuries to calm frazzled nerves. In Western medicine reserpine is widely prescribed in low doses to relieve high blood pressure. But it occasionally has an unfortunate side effect—profound depression.

The other drug was a tuberculosis remedy called isoniazid. Among its side effects is an ability to elevate mood and induce a sense of overall contentment. And what if both drugs are administered together? The best of both worlds, it seems, for the patient calms down while his outlook remains sunny. As researchers studied the biochemistry of the two drugs, they found that both affect the brain's supply of two key neurotransmitters, serotonin and noradrenaline. These two neurotransmitters have a very complex—and not yet fully understood—relationship. Noradrenaline is generated mostly in the midbrain, in a small cluster of bluish cells called the locus coeruleus. But while these cells are not numerous, their branches extend throughout the limbic system, back into the cerebellum and up through the neocortex. In discharging their supply of noradrenaline, they promote an attitude of alertness, pleasure and excitement. They must achieve a delicate balance, however. It is thought that too much noradrenaline causes agitation and stress; too little may mean depression.

The same may be true of serotonin. Emanating from a nearby midbrain cell group called the raphe nuclei, serotonin regulates such factors as sleepiness, body temperature and sensory perception. When deficient, it too may produce depression. The complicated action of these two transmitters in the brain's synapses depends on the presence of still another chemical, a brain and liver enzyme called monoamine oxidase. It is the job of MAO to break down excess amounts of serotonin and noradrenaline. Various antidepressant drugs try to correct any imbalance of noradrenaline and serotonin by either inhibiting MAO so that it does not destroy too much of the neurotransmitters, or by decreasing some of the receptors for noradrenaline and

Love's Elixir

Infatuation—at least when it is described clinically—sounds like a diagnosis of manic psychosis. Thinking is irrational, replete with sweeping generalizations, unsubstantiated claims and illogical predictions. Mood is altered, leaving love's captive highly energetic, optimistic, hungry to communicate. These are also the symptoms of an amphetamine high.

Some scientists suggest that a romantic crush may affect neurotransmission in a similar way to amphetamines. Such stimulants trigger the release of dopamine and, even more importantly, they extend the normal period of time that dopamine remains in the synaptic cleft. This affects the emotional centers in the brain and puts the individual in a hyper state of euphoria. The mystique of a new, intriguing person, coupled with fantasies of endless future adoration and compatibility, is believed to alter brain chemistry by triggering "love transmitters."

Noradrenaline and dopamine are possible candidates, though this remains a matter of speculation. Clearer evidence exists for a love-endorphin connection. Endorphins, the brain's natural opiates, appear instrumental in the calm feelings of security associated with long-term attachment, after the kite-like highs of being "in love" flutter down to earth. The pain of separation is attributed to withdrawal from a steady supply of endorphins.

Hormones also are thought to play leading roles in love, especially in motivating sex. Research, mostly with animals, shows that hormones in sweat, called pheromones, act as aphrodisiacs to light up emotion centers in the limbic system, which is connected to the pathway of smell.

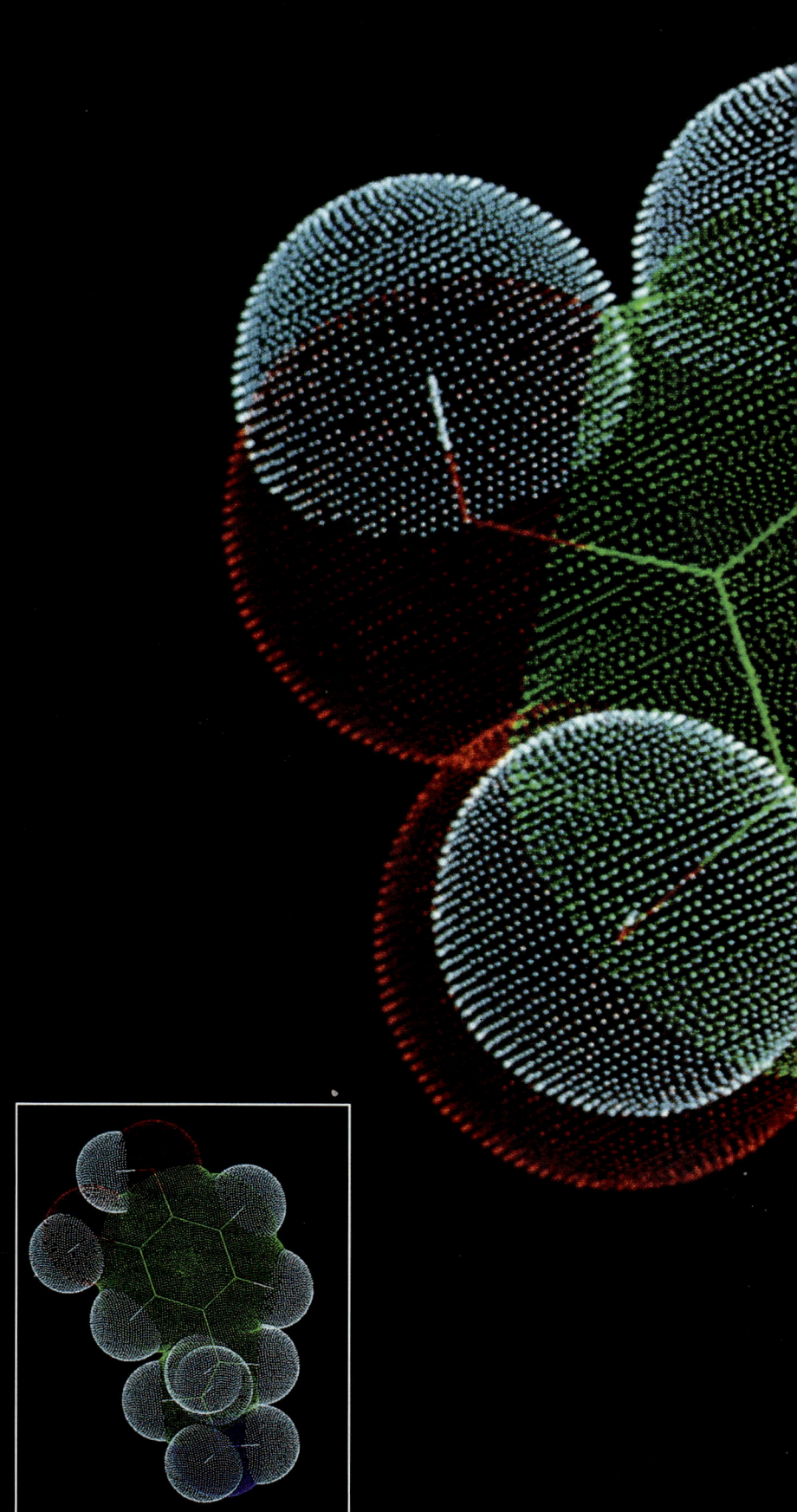

In redefining the "chemistry of love," scientists are studying computer-generated images of neurotransmitters. This noradrenaline molecule looks like a tumultuous burst of fireworks coloring a night sky. Inset is a similar image of dopamine, also suspected of being one of Cupid's arrows.

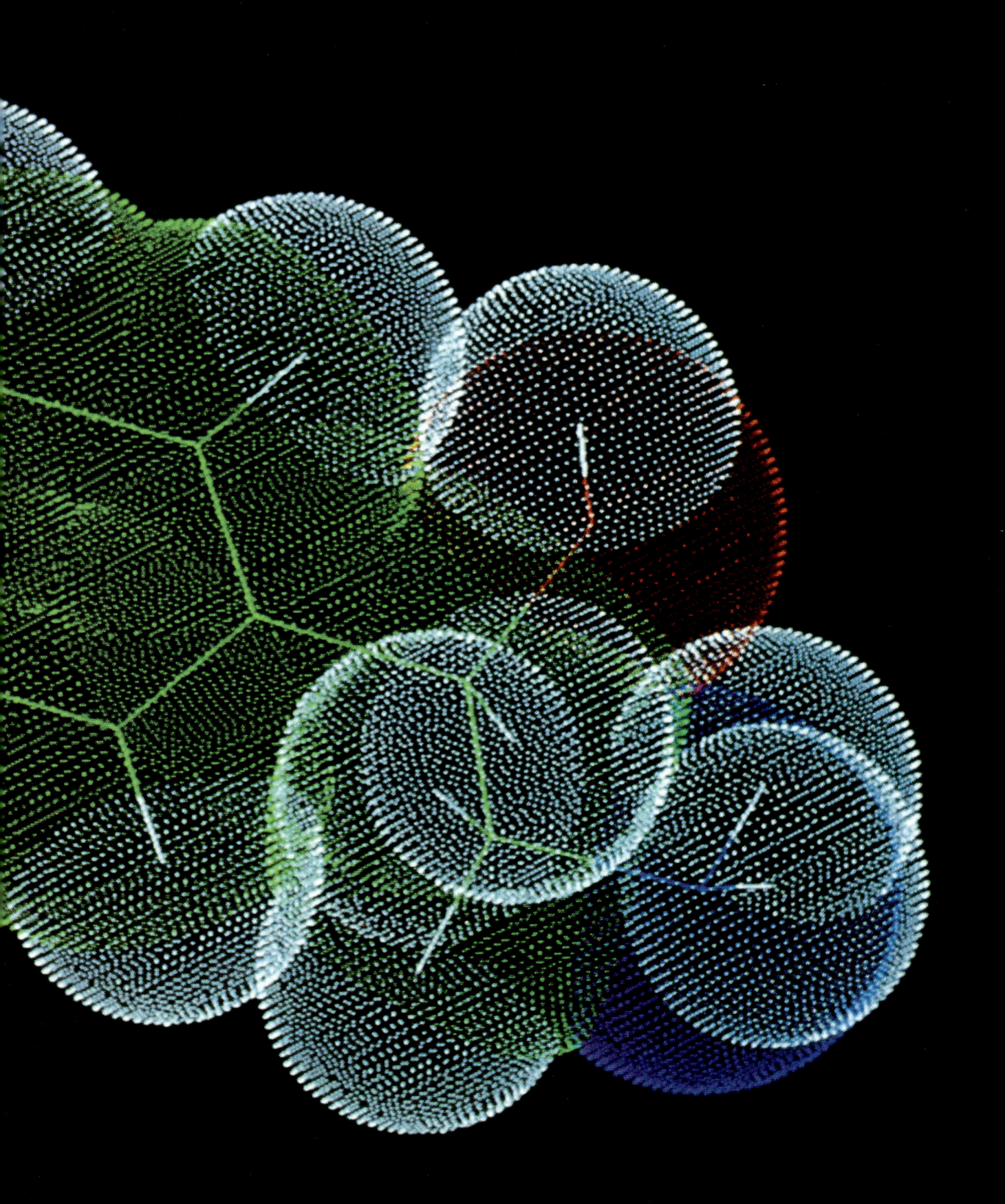

serotonin. Other treatments increase the transmission of serotonin or block the reuptake of the two neurotransmitters.

With the pharmacopeia now available, it would seem that science has all but conquered the problem of mood disorders. But depression has many neurological causes—and any number of psychiatric ones—and in some cases drugs do not work. One common mood disorder attacks only in winter. Its victims—who may number as many as 20 percent of residents in some far northern countries where winter nights are very long—become sluggish and irritable as the days grow short. A few become deeply withdrawn. Then, as the sun returns, they perk up, their energy surges and they function normally again.

This syndrome of winter blues, called seasonal affective disorder, or SAD, relates directly to the hours of daylight in each 24-hour period. The explanation for it lies, in part, in the hormone melatonin, a secretion of the pineal gland. Melatonin is a natural sedative, which slows down the rhythms of the body. It induces sleep when the sun goes down, and as winter approaches it prompts animals that hibernate to seek out their lairs. In people with the syndrome, melatonin brings on a kind of emotional winter hibernation.

The cure—short of moving south each year when the snow flies—is to lengthen the day by artificial means. One method is to treat the victim to a daily dose of high-intensity, full-spectrum light, which mimics the rays of the sun. Hormones thus fooled, the SAD sufferer generally recovers within the week.

Beyond light therapy for SAD people, and drug treatment for other forms of depression, there is a continuing need for traditional forms of psychotherapy. Mood swings so engrain themselves in the circuits of thought and memory that even

MENTAL ILLNESS

Statistics show that almost one in every eight people consults his doctor at some time for problems that are primarily psychological. The chart below shows the lifetime risk of developing various mental disorders. Women outnumber men by about two to one in the category of neurotic disorders—feelings and thoughts that most people experience at some time but which, if persistent and severe, can lead to a nervous breakdown. Men and women suffer equally from the more serious psychotic illnesses such as schizophrenia.

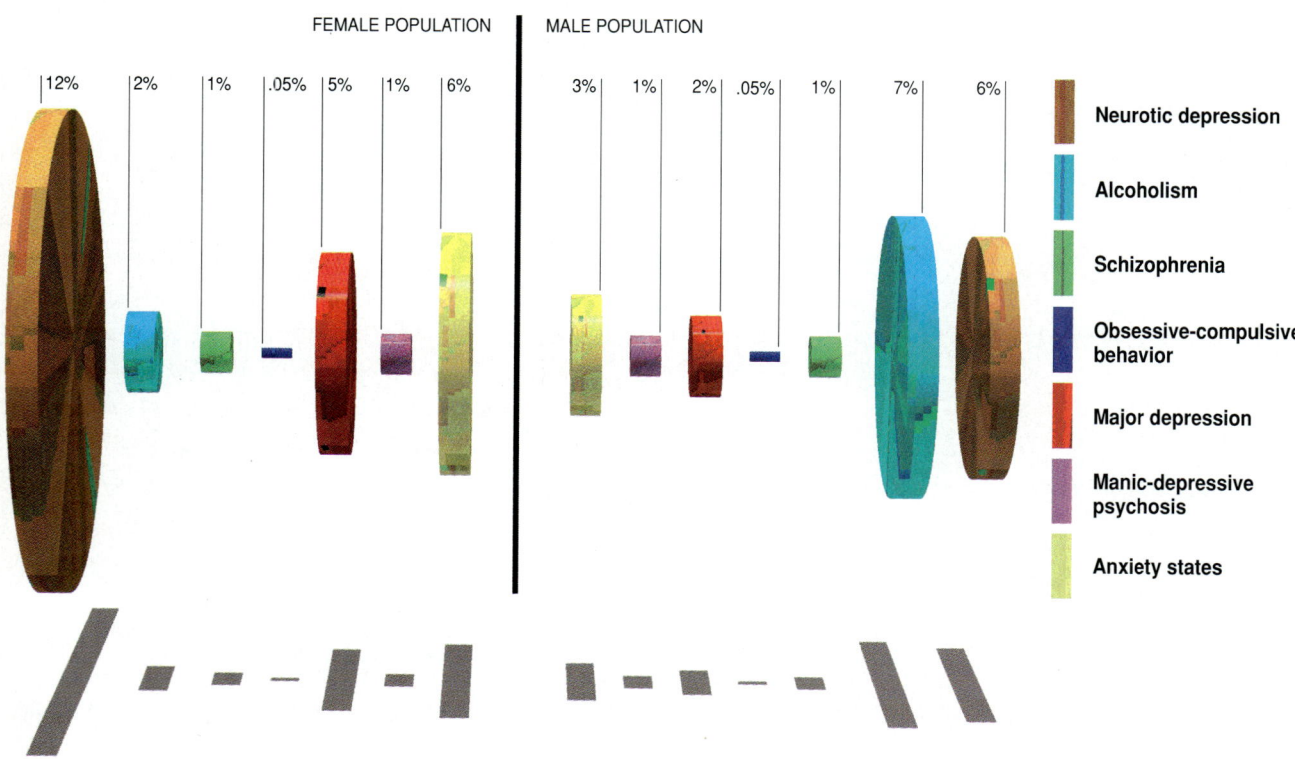

MOOD, MOLECULES AND MADNESS

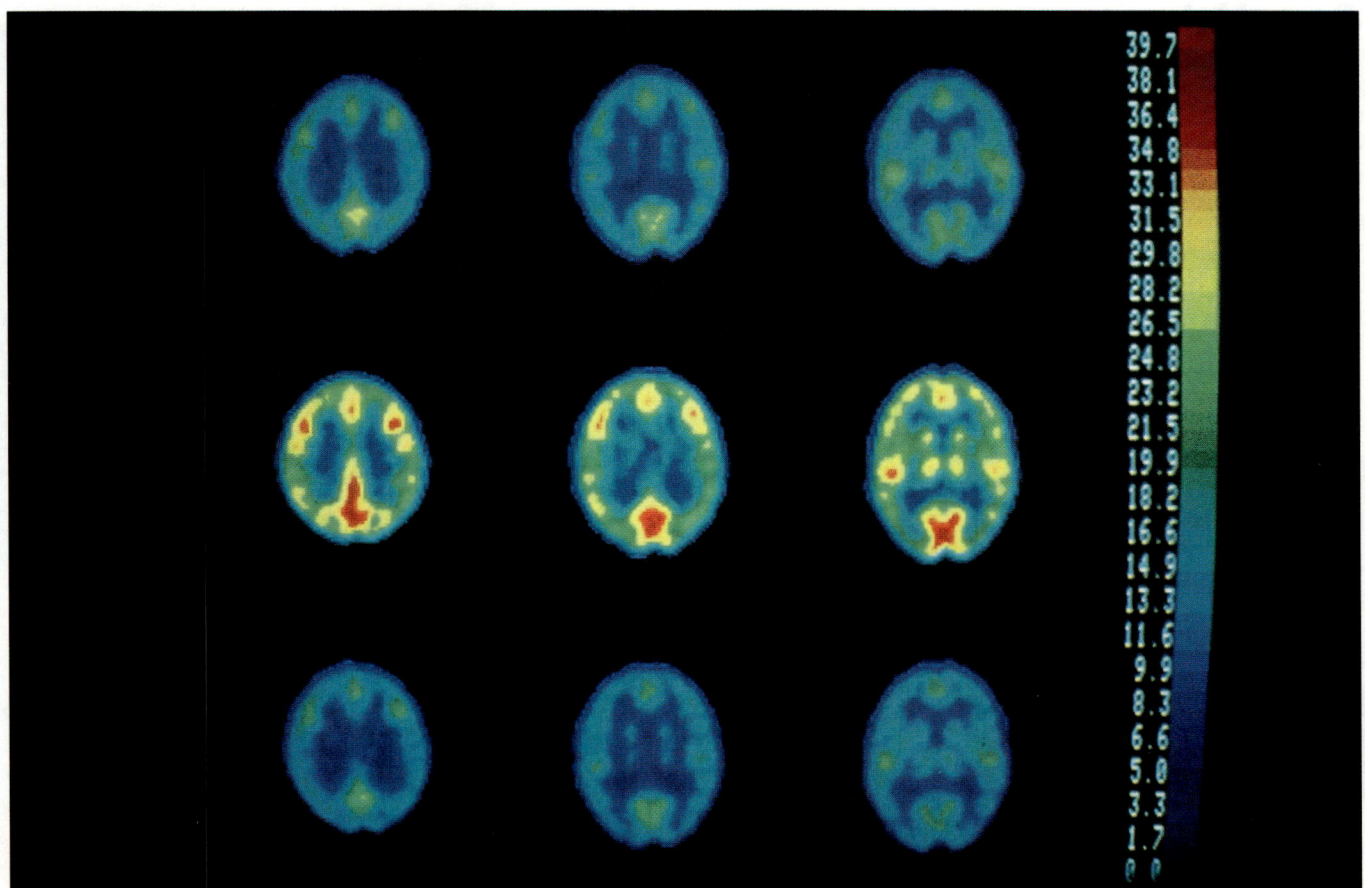

These PET scans monitor the radical swings of electrochemical energy in the brain of a manic-depressive patient who is going from depression to mania to depression again in 48-hour cycles. The blue of the top row of scans aptly portrays depression. The red and yellow of the center row of scans, taken one day later, show high glucose consumption rates, indicating manic activity. By the following day, the rapid-cycling patient is depressed again.

when they cease, the patient may be left bewildered and non-functional. "Which me is *me*?" asked one recovering manic-depressive. "The wild, impulsive, chaotic, energetic and crazy one? Or the shy, withdrawn, desperate, suicidal, doomed and tired one?" Only long sessions with a psychiatrist would provide the answer.

One ailment that continues to baffle both psychiatrists and neurologists is the crippling affliction known as schizophrenia. Its victims account for perhaps 50 percent of all admissions to mental hospitals, and 10 to 15 percent of them remain there for life. Even Freud believed there was no hope of a psychiatric cure. The unpredictable, chameleon-like disease may strike without warning, grab hold for a short time and then let go, never to return. Or it may settle in for good, condemning its prey to a life of perpetual madness. Some patients may be hostile and agitated, storming about in tantrums of gusty emotion. Others become passive to the point of immobility, and retreat into a shadow world of internal terrors. Many hallucinate, hearing voices and seeing objects that do not exist. Thoughts become jumbled and associations bizarre; some patients claim to be someone else. Often two contradictory ideas occur at the same moment, and the patient accepts both of them. People suffering from schizophrenia may believe that the doctors and families who are trying to help them are attempting to kill them.

One common thread runs through all cases: Ideas and emotions have no apparent connection. In schizophrenia—the term means "divided brain"—the patient is cut off from his own feelings and the feelings of others. It is almost as though some psychic scalpel had severed the pathways between his limbic system and

STRESS SCALE

Occupations that involve tough mental and emotional challenges—responsibility for human life, control of enormous sums of money, hair-raising deadlines—conjure up images of ulcers and nervous breakdowns. While this may be true, there is another trap lying at the other end of the continuum—the stress-laden boredom of a profession that provides very little stimulation and job satisfaction. Statistics show that this kind of stress is just as damaging as the other.

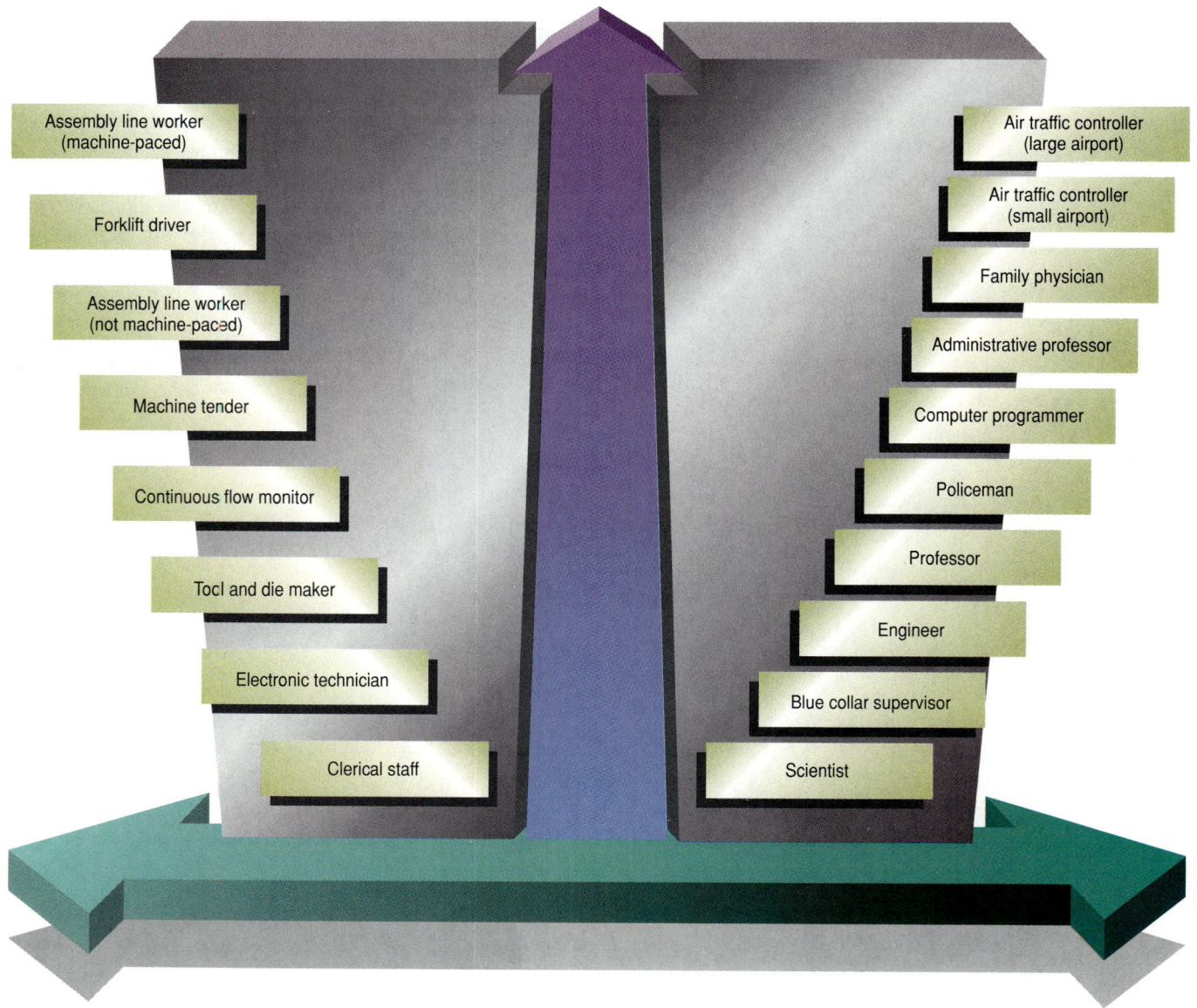

his cortex. "I felt a cleavage in my mind—as if my brain had split," wrote Emily Dickinson many decades before the condition had been medically defined. "I tried to match it—seam by seam—but could not make them fit."

One of the tragedies of schizophrenia is that it most often attacks the young. The onset almost always occurs before the age of 35, and frequently strikes in adolescence. It also tends to run in families. In the general population, one person in a hundred comes down with the ailment; but if a blood relative has schizophrenia, the risk of developing the ailment is 14 times higher. In the case of identical twins, the odds are nearly 50-50. The implication is that schizophrenia's cause is partly genetic. Some defect in the genes may disrupt the brain, causing a deterioration in its structure, or creating a biochemical imbalance that renders an individual more vulnerable to psychological or psychosocial stresses and which can result in mental chaos.

One likely culprit is the neurotransmitter dopamine. A multipurpose agent related chemically to noradrenaline, dopamine is essential for controlling complex bodily movements; death of dopamine neurons in the substantia nigra results in the persistent tremors of Parkinson's disease. It also plays a role in governing emotions. Emanating from two midbrain sites, the substantia nigra and the ventral tegmental area, its pathways meander through the limbic system, and also into the frontal lobe of the cortex, the seat of conscious thought. In explaining schizophrenia one theory postulates that there is an overabundance of dopamine in certain cortical and limbic areas.

If an excess of dopamine is somehow connected with schizophrenia, could the symptoms be treated by blocking the postsynaptic receptors? The answer is a qualified yes. Chlorpromazine, a tranquilizing drug often prescribed to overcome anxiety and agitation in mental illness, also seems to work with patients in the acute, hallucinatory phase of schizophrenia. Delusions cease, agitation diminishes and reason returns. Because of it, thousands of patients have been able to leave psychiatric hospitals and lead reasonably normal lives.

No one knows quite why this works—or even how the dopamine pathways go awry. It may be that the neurons simply secrete too much of the neurotransmitter. But there are other possibilities. Schizophrenic patients may have more dopamine receptors than normal, or the ones they have may be overly sensitive. Or it may be that the mechanisms that sop up excess dopamine, or that break it down, are faulty. Nor can it be said that the dopamine itself is a cause of schizophrenia. The transmitter's unusual abundance may be merely a byproduct of some more basic process—perhaps even of the disordered thoughts and fantasies of the disease itself. And chlorpromazine is no final cure. It simply helps alleviate some of the symptoms.

STRESSED OUT

One type of psychic malaise is so common that people tend to view it as a normal condition of modern life. We live in an age of stress. Evidence can be seen in the rising executive who burns out in midcareer, in the war veteran and his recurring nightmares, in statistics for ulcers and heart attacks. It is no coincidence that the three most widely prescribed kinds of drugs today are ulcer compounds, blood pressure medication and tranquilizers.

Simply stated, stress is any condition or event that puts extra demands on the body. Some stress is physically induced—a sharp pain, for example, or the nagging frustration of loud, persistent noise. A broken leg is physically stressful, as the body rallies its resources to repair the damage. Other forms of stress—the pressures of work, or a family argument—are clearly psychological. No single event so strains the system as the emotional trauma of a loved one's death, or of a divorce.

Physiologically, the common responses to all these types of stress appear to be activation of the sympathetic nervous system, the hypothalamus, pituitary and adrenal glands. Consider the most basic type of stress scenario—a sudden emergency such as an impending car crash. The entire organism is galvanized into a state of maximum readiness. It is the classic fight-or-flight response, prompted by the quick release of noradrenaline—also known as norepinephrine—and other stress-related transmitters. The adrenal medullae secrete adrenaline, or epinephrine, and noradrenaline into general circulation. The sympathetic system also contributes noradrenaline so that the body is primed and ready to respond.

At the same time another transmitter system also comes into play, and this one tends to moderate the response. On signal from the hypothalamus, the pituitary

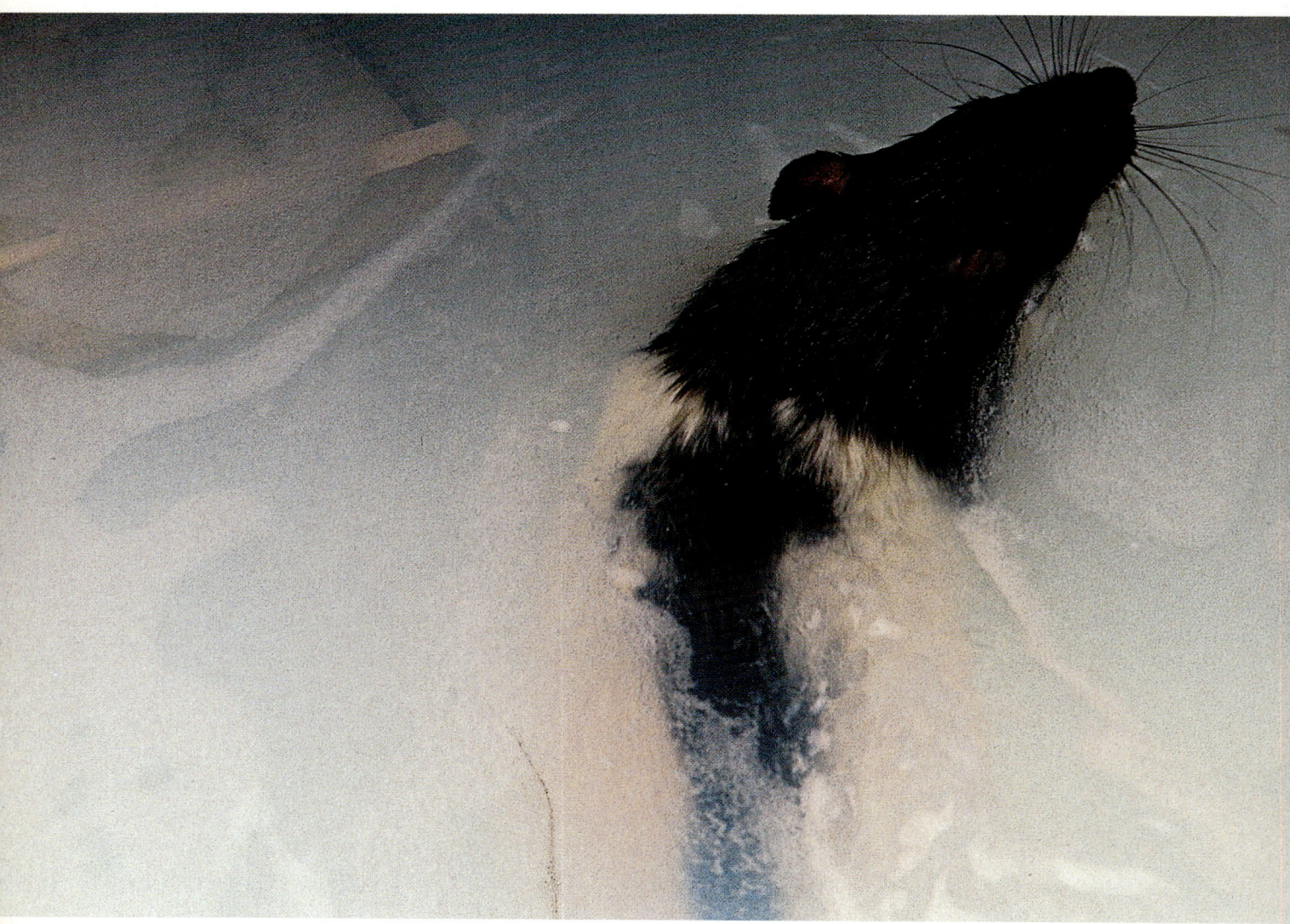

This test rat, swimming in water made opaque by the addition of powdered milk so that it can no longer see the pool's resting platform through the water, has forgotten the location of the platform following damage to its hippocampus. Experiments with rats indicate that stress may harm neurons essential for memory. Rats who respond poorly to stress show damage to their hippocampal neurons, possibly as a result of a continual bombardment of stress-related hormones.

secretes the neurohormone adrenocorticotropin (ACTH), which in turn triggers a second adrenal response. Out pours the hormone cortisol, which feeds back to the pituitary and the hypothalamus, telling them to shut off their stimulation. Cortisol has other functions as well. It raises the glucose level in the blood, providing extra energy for the brain. By promoting the breakdown of protein, it frees the amino acids needed to repair cellular damage. And it raises blood pressure.

Because cortisol is easily detected in the blood, scientists use it to help assess the degree of stress in various situations. Paratroopers, training for their first jump, have high levels of blood cortisol. Then, as the jumps become routine, the cortisol level declines. Far less hazardous prospects than leaping from an airplane will also generate large quantities of cortisol. Simply climbing aboard a passenger jet does it for some people. So may speaking in public, entering a tennis match, running for a bus or shopping for Christmas presents.

These situations may not be inherently dangerous or distasteful, nor is stress itself necessarily a harmful thing. In some people, the emotional jolt that the stress response provides is almost a biological necessity, mobilizing the body to peak performance. Without some stress, life would be intolerably bland. The sky diver, the mountain climber, the financier striving to close a deal, are each motivated, in part, by the adrenaline rush such activity brings.

For these individuals, according to Dr. Joel Elkes of Johns Hopkins Medical School in Maryland, "extreme stress produces a pleasurable arousal, followed by a feeling of release." The presence of noradrenaline, combined with the boost in blood sugar, rivets the attention on the task at hand. Extraneous thoughts and sensations tend to disappear. Other transmitters block the sensation of pain—which may explain why a football player can break a bone and still finish the game without being aware that he has been injured. At the same time, the ability to absorb information is often enhanced. The brain structure most closely associated with the translation of items in short-term memory into long-term memory, the hippocampus, is densely populated with cortisol receptors.

The problems arise when stress persists or becomes so intense it cannot be controlled. Under these conditions stress may soon turn into distress, as its initial benefits reverse themselves. Short-term memory is impaired; the ability to perform declines. The nervous system loses its attentive edge. Exhaustion sets in. The victim feels emotionally numb, and succumbs to a sense of apathy and defeat. A state of clinical depression may follow. Patients suffering from depressive disorders often show the same high cortisol levels that characterize chronic stress.

Cortisol has a number of long-term ill effects. If maintained at excessive levels, it upsets the body's normal protein balance. Blood pressure remains unhealthily elevated. Too much cortisol destroys neurons in the hippocampus. Furthermore, it has a profound effect on the immune system, seriously impeding the body's ability to fight disease.

The link between states of mind and immune response is difficult to track, but there are indications that it is a close relationship. Immune cells are known to have receptors for various hormones and neurotransmitters, including noradrenaline, ACTH and cortisol. Immune cells both receive messages from and send messages to the brain. Several studies have shown that electrical stimulation of the hypothalamus can promote an immune response, while a surgical cut in the same area will dampen it. In one experiment, rats were injected with cells that triggered their immune systems and the neurons in their brains—a clear indication that "the brain actually knew what the immune system was doing," according to Dr. Hugo Besedovsky of the Swiss Research Institute, who conducted the procedure. Given this close correspondence, it is not surprising that people under prolonged stress are highly vulnerable to colds, fevers and other ailments.

Not everyone is affected to the same degree—indeed, some people seem to thrive on stress. Meeting a challenge with confidence and skill, their noradrenaline flows, but their cortisol level stays low. A major factor appears to be control: The more authority an individual wields over a situation, the less harm it does him.

Dramatic demonstration of this phenomenon can be seen in another experiment with laboratory rats. Three groups of rats were put in adjacent cages. One group continued to lead uneventful rodent lives. Another group was subjected to a series of mild but unpredictable electric shocks. The third group also received the shock treatment, but could stop the current by turning a small wheel. After some weeks of this regimen, biopsies were performed. Rats from the passive second group, which had no control over the shocks, were riddled with gastric ulcers. The rats with the cut-off wheel had fewer ulcers, while the shock-free, test-control rats had no problem with ulcers.

Humans, apparently, react the same way. To an outsider, it seems that no job could be more stressful and ulcer-producing than managing a large corporation. But in a 1974 survey, top-ranking executives in major companies proved to be far healthier and more worry-free than the general population. Their mortality rate was 37 percent lower than that of other men in the same age group. Stress took a much greater toll on middle-management executives, who bore heavy responsibilities but wielded less power. Worse off still were factory workers, forced to meet the rigid demands of the production line while deprived of the benefits and satisfactions enjoyed by their bosses. The secret, according to the experts, is not to avoid stress, but to enjoy and be good at one's life work.

Some forms of stress are more severe. Terrifying panic attacks—recurring episodes of sudden, acute anxiety that often strike without warning, and for no apparent reason—cripple an estimated 2 to 5 percent of the population. The palms sweat, knees turn to jelly, the heart palpitates, the breath comes in gasps, if it comes at all. There is often a feeling of vertigo, and perhaps hot and cold flashes. Most frightening of all is an eerie sense of unreality. "I feel I'm in another world," is how one victim described it. "I know I'm there, but I'm really not." This severe depersonalization is not entirely understood. One theory holds that the attacks are brought on by a dysfunction of the system mediating GABA, a neurotransmitter that inhibits neural activity and allows neurons to receive new information in an orderly manner. Other neurotransmitters have been implicated in panic disorders, which are thought to be linked to major depression.

In some cases, panic attacks may result from the unconscious memory of some buried emotional shock, a phenomenon known as post-traumatic stress disorder. Front-line veterans returning from war often experience it, and so may the victims of rape or physical assault. Studies have shown that a single instance of overwhelming terror may cause permanent changes in brain chemistry, making the individual abnormally vulnerable to later stressful incidents. One theory is that cells in the locus coeruleus, which produces noradrenaline, remain hyperactive. The same may apply to the hypothalamus and the amygdala, which then would continue to alert both body and emotions for an emergency that no longer existed.

Closely akin to panic are various phobias. One out of every eight adults is plagued by some bugbear of anxiety, whether it be a fear of spiders, snakes, heights or large crowds. An almost universal phobia is stage fright. Pre-curtain anxiety can propel a performer to lofty heights of artistic expression, but too much of it can be disastrous.

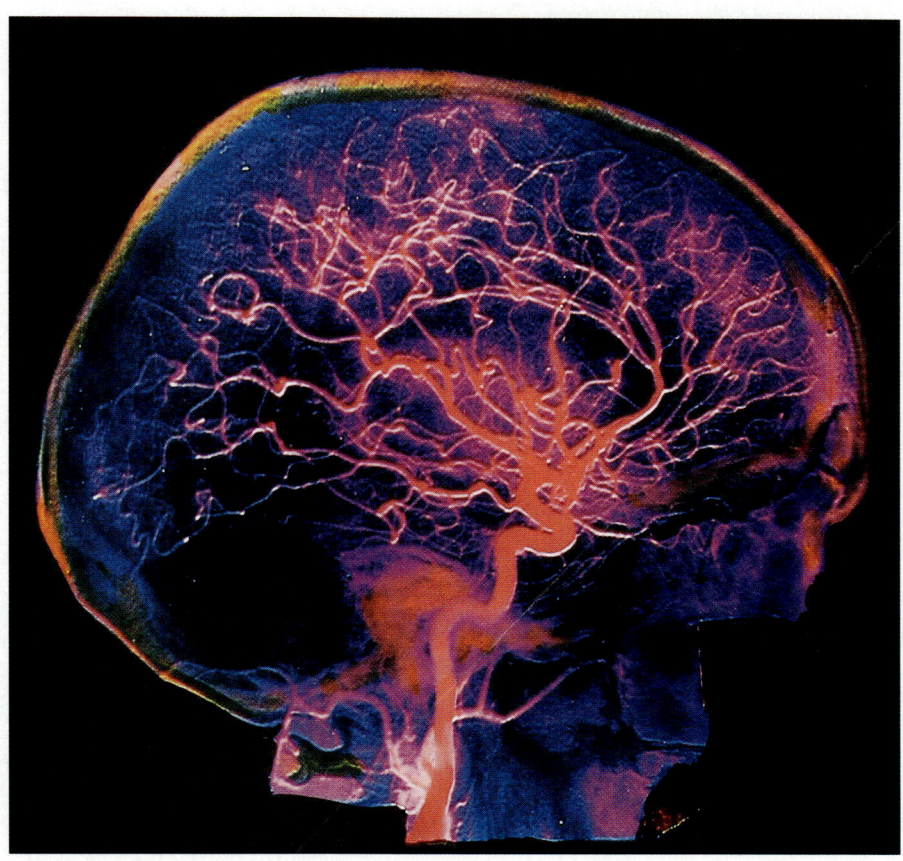

An extensive network of blood vessels crisscrosses the brain like a well-plotted transportation system. As well as feeding the brain with oxygen and glucose, blood vessels serve as hormone pipelines. The pituitary, chief gland of the endocrine system, uses blood-borne hormones to communicate with other glands.

As in any stressful situation, the best remedy is to establish firm and competent control. To this end, actors rehearse and pianists practice. People with phobias can often learn, through work with a psychotherapist, to confront their fears and overcome them. The recurring anxieties of post-traumatic stress disorder may also give way to cognitive therapy.

One method for coping with stress is to think through a challenging situation in advance, visualizing each step. Champion golfer Jack Nicklaus maintains that he never hits a shot, even in practice, without having a sharp, in-focus picture of it in his head. A vital part of the image is watching the ball drop into the hole. It may be that habituation to the thought of success quiets the hyperactivity of the adrenaline and cortisol secreting pathways, thus making success possible.

Various drugs also relieve anxiety, at least temporarily. The problem of stage fright has been treated with so-called beta blockers, a type of heart medication that binds to the neural receptors for adrenaline. The beta blockers have less effect

Put on a Happy Face

Pop psychology axioms extolling the salutary effects of acting cheery and bright often sound so shallow that it is easy to shrug them off as childishly facile. However, neuropsychologists suggest that the feedback loop linking the brain's mood centers to receptors throughout the body support formulas such as: "Act happy, and you will feel happy." Meanwhile, experts on brain chemistry and the immune system are confident that laughter is good not only for the soul, but for the body as well.

Facial expression, posture, the speed and precision of movement—all are barometers of an individual's emotional state. This relationship depends on a constant flow of electrochemical signals from the limbic system—the team of brain structures regulating mood—to the body. But information flows from body to brain as well, bodily "symptoms" providing data upon which the limbic system updates mood. Just as a glum demeanor perpetuates a vicious circle of brain and body infusing each other with negativity, manifestations of happiness can

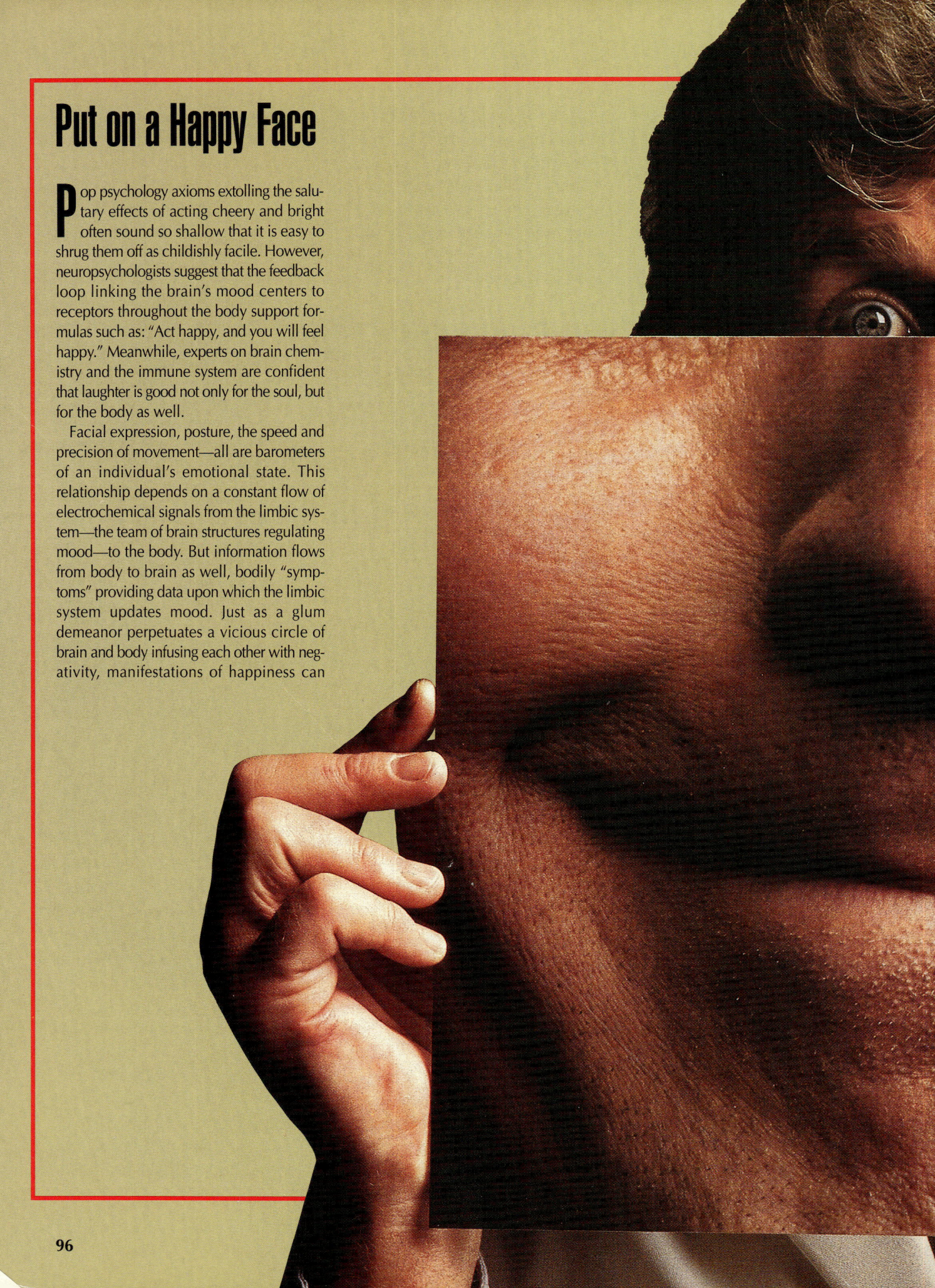

MOOD, MOLECULES AND MADNESS

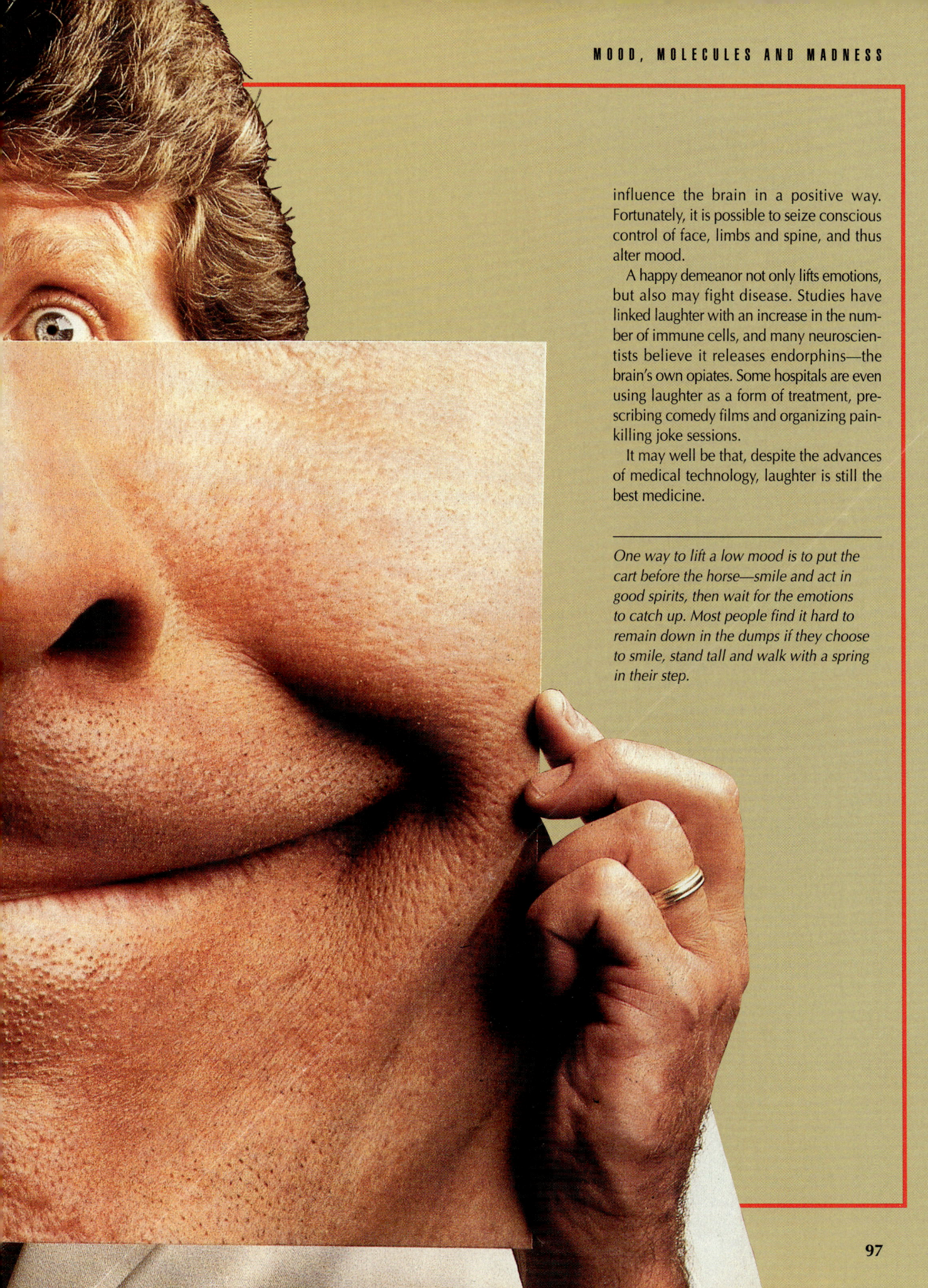

influence the brain in a positive way. Fortunately, it is possible to seize conscious control of face, limbs and spine, and thus alter mood.

A happy demeanor not only lifts emotions, but also may fight disease. Studies have linked laughter with an increase in the number of immune cells, and many neuroscientists believe it releases endorphins—the brain's own opiates. Some hospitals are even using laughter as a form of treatment, prescribing comedy films and organizing pain-killing joke sessions.

It may well be that, despite the advances of medical technology, laughter is still the best medicine.

One way to lift a low mood is to put the cart before the horse—smile and act in good spirits, then wait for the emotions to catch up. Most people find it hard to remain down in the dumps if they choose to smile, stand tall and walk with a spring in their step.

97

on noradrenaline, however, so the performer remains fully alert, mentally primed for the event ahead but free from the bodily tensions of an overexcited autonomic nervous system. Diazepam (known more commonly by its trade name, Valium) and other related compounds also have an anti-anxiety effect by enhancing the calming action of the neurotransmitter GABA.

The difficulty with some drugs is that they can become habit-forming. A more natural antidote to stress is exercise. All the primordial circuits of fight or flight have evolved to mobilize the organism toward a single end—intense physical activity. Exercise provides the intended release. It also brings its own neural pleasures in the form of yet another type of neurotransmitter: the endorphins.

HOOKING THE BRAIN

Endorphins are natural painkillers released in the brain during moments of stress. They may explain why a marathon runner, subjecting his body to excruciating punishment, feels a sense of elation as he clocks off the miles. Neuroscientists believe any number of stimuli may trigger endorphin release—music, laughter, chocolate cake or chili peppers, or even a good cry over a sentimental movie.

Back in the early 1970s, a number of scientists were searching to explain why morphine and other derivatives of the opium poppy have such a powerful effect on the nervous system. Long used by doctors to relieve pain, the opiates promote feelings of contentment, detachment, lassitude and freedom from distress. Some work their magic in remarkably minute doses. Such potency suggested that the opiates have an immediate transmission route to the brain.

Experiments using radioactively tagged opiates confirmed the theory. What is more, the opiates plug directly into certain key receptors in the limbic area. But why should the brain, in the course of its long evolution, have developed receptors for the juice of one particular poppy plant?

Two researchers in Aberdeen, Scotland, supplied part of the answer. In quest of a new painkiller, Dr. Hans Kosterlitz and Dr. John Hughes examined pig brains and found that they contained a substance whose effects were similar to morphine. They called the new material *enkephalin*—Greek for "in the head"— and proceeded to test its pain-relieving properties. The results were disappointing. Enkephalin is only mildly effective as a painkiller. Nonetheless, they had discovered something of major importance—that the brain itself produces a kind of morphine. Further answers would come from the work of C. Li, a neurochemist at the University of California. About a decade earlier Li had been examining secretions of the pituitary gland, hoping to find an enzyme that controls the metabolism of fats. He had decided to work with camel pituitaries and asked one of his students, an Iraqi, to bring him some. The student returned from summer vacation with 500 dried camel pituitaries. They held no fat enzyme, but they were chock full of a mysterious compound that Li had never before encountered. He saved some for future explorations.

When Li heard about the work of the two Scottish researchers, the news struck him with the force of revelation. Enkephalin, he realized, must be one of the molec-

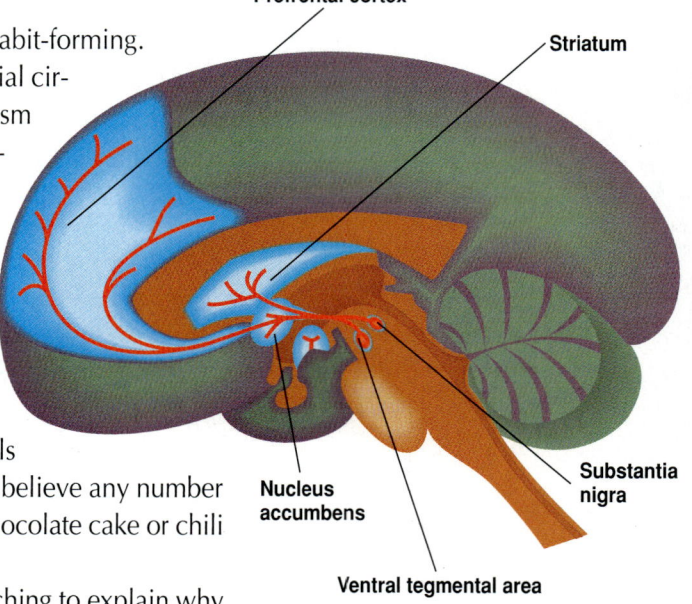

PATHWAYS OF DOPAMINE

Important circuits of the neurotransmitter dopamine originate from the ventral tegmental area and the substantia nigra and make stops in the nucleus accumbens, striatum and the prefrontal cortex. A second cousin of the drugs ice (a type of amphetamine) and crack (a smokable form of cocaine), dopamine mediates various brain functions, including movement and emotion.

MOOD, MOLECULES AND MADNESS

ular building blocks in his mysterious compound. What he had discovered almost 10 years earlier was beta-endorphin, the brain's natural opiate. (The word endorphin is, in fact, an abridgement of the term endogenous morphine-like substance.) Injected into the brains of test animals, beta-endorphin is 48 times more powerful than morphine itself.

Both the endorphins and the enkephalins—each has several molecular varieties—are part of the body's defense against pain. The enkephalins are not addictive because they are destroyed rapidly by enzymes as soon as they act at receptors. They shut off the sharp, sudden stab that occurs from a pinprick, say, or from the touch of a hot iron. Produced mostly by the pituitary gland, the endorphins help moderate the deep-seated ache that persists over time. Opiate receptors, into which the endorphins fit, are highly concentrated in many of the limbic structures, including the septum and amygdala.

No wonder, then, that the endorphins bring pleasure. Nor is it surprising that people become hooked on opiates. Opium, and its derivatives morphine and heroin, are artificial neurotransmitters; racing to the limbic synapses, they mimic the brain's own natural high. The faster they find their way to the brain, the higher their intrinsic addictiveness—which is why injecting a drug, or sniffing or smoking it, is the addict's preferred technique. But taken in this manner, the drug becomes doubly addictive.

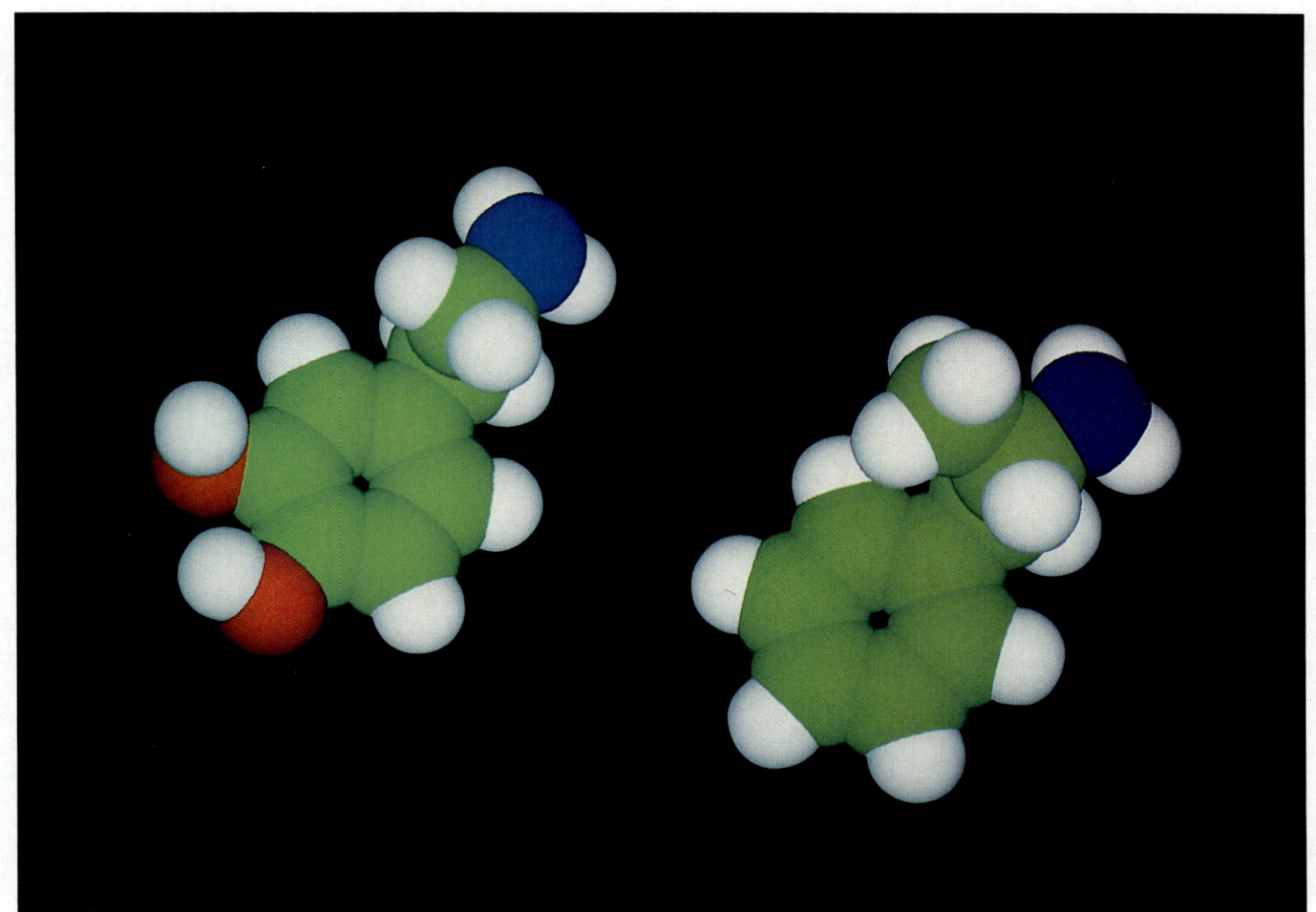

The subtle structural difference between the drug amphetamine (right) and the natural neurotransmitter dopamine (left) permits amphetamine to operate as a "false transmitter." Amphetamine promotes dopamine release by partially mimicking dopamine at key sites in the dopamine neuron. Many drugs, including prescription medications, interact with the brain because their molecular structures resemble those of the brain's neurotransmitters.

Only part of the opiates' hold is the pleasure they bring, however. The brain adapts quickly to neural stimuli, and chronic administration of narcotics causes changes in its chemistry. The secretion of natural opiates declines, their job having been taken over by the drug. Dependence occurs when the drug is required to function normally and when there are symptoms if the drug is withdrawn. Withdrawal symptoms can be alleviated by taking another dose of the drug. And thus starts the vicious circle. As the user's tolerance rises, he needs increasing doses to achieve the desired drug effect. Addiction, then, is defined as this state of dependence produced by the habitual taking of a certain drug.

Denied his required fix, the addict goes through a period of agonizing withdrawal. Within hours after his last shot of heroin, for example, he begins to sneeze and sweat, his eyes water and his muscles ache. Then, for the next 36 to 72 hours, he may be hit by muscle spasms, cramps, heart palpitations, vomiting and diarrhea. In a years-old debate, researchers are still divided over the question of whether the motivation for continued drug use comes from an attempt to avoid withdrawal symptoms or the lure of drug-related pleasure.

Many types of drugs are abused—marijuana, amphetamines, hallucinogens such as LSD, tranquilizers and antidepressants are only a few of the most commonly abused. The two most devastating, in terms of the number of people affected, are alcohol and tobacco. Each casts its spell, in part, by affecting one or more of the limbic neurotransmitter systems. And most drugs, when abused, carry the risk of serious dependency.

The most rapidly addictive substance in current use is cocaine, particularly when it is smoked in the form of crack. The high it induces is swift and bracing—a sudden euphoric rush that explodes in the brain within 15 seconds of the first puff. The user feels confident and alert, his thoughts flowing quickly and with the illusion of utmost clarity. Even if naturally shy, he now finds himself witty and outgoing, brimming with sex appeal and on top of the world. But the euphoria is of very short duration—a drug may be metabolized in five to fifteen minutes. The high can depart almost as abruptly as it arrived, leaving the user strangely despondent and searching for another hit.

Cocaine's attraction is thought to be mediated through its interaction with the dopamine circuits. In addition to the receptors that allow transmission of the electrochemical signal from a dopamine neuron to another neuron, there are molecular uptake sites on the dopamine neuron that terminate the action of dopamine by taking it back up into the dopamine nerve terminal. Cocaine blocks these reuptake sites. As a result, the dopamine concentrations build in the synapse. A similar effect occurs with a related class of drugs, the amphetamines, which also may increase the release of dopamine by interfering with its storage inside the cell. Amphetamines produce a similar kind of ebullient high.

Much of both drugs' effects occur in a region of the limbic system known as the nucleus accumbens, where a large number of dopamine axons terminate. The abuse of either cocaine or amphetamines may do some permanent neurological damage. Chronic administration in test animals has produced permanent damage, but the results in humans are still being investigated. At its worst, though, the outcome is a psychotic condition similar to schizophrenia, which is thought to be a dopamine-related syndrome.

MOOD, MOLECULES AND MADNESS

NATURAL (ENDORPHIN)

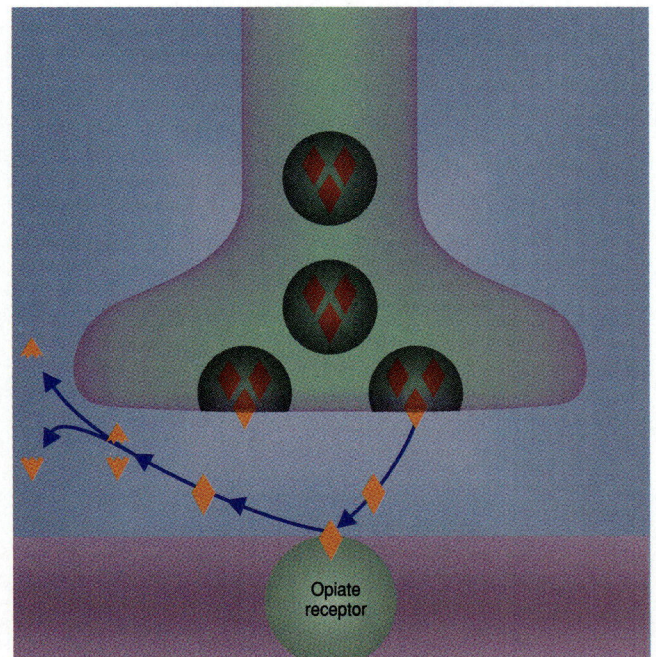

CHEMICAL (MORPHINE)

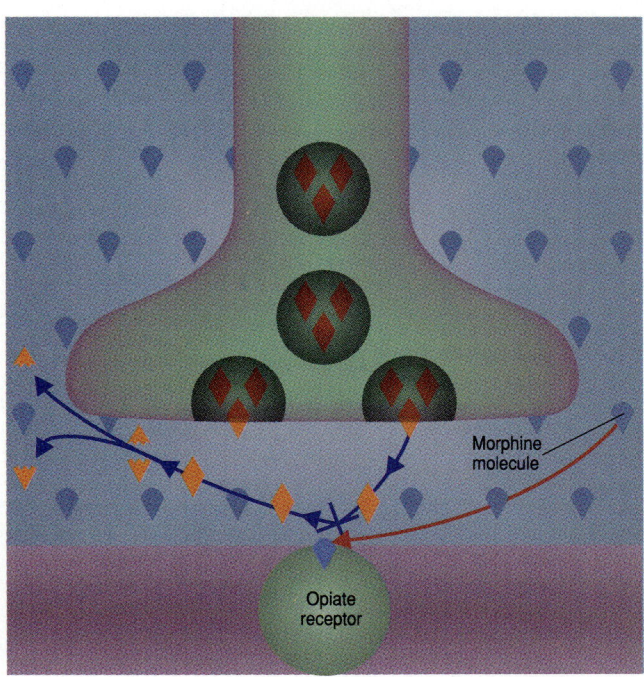

NATURAL (DOPAMINE)

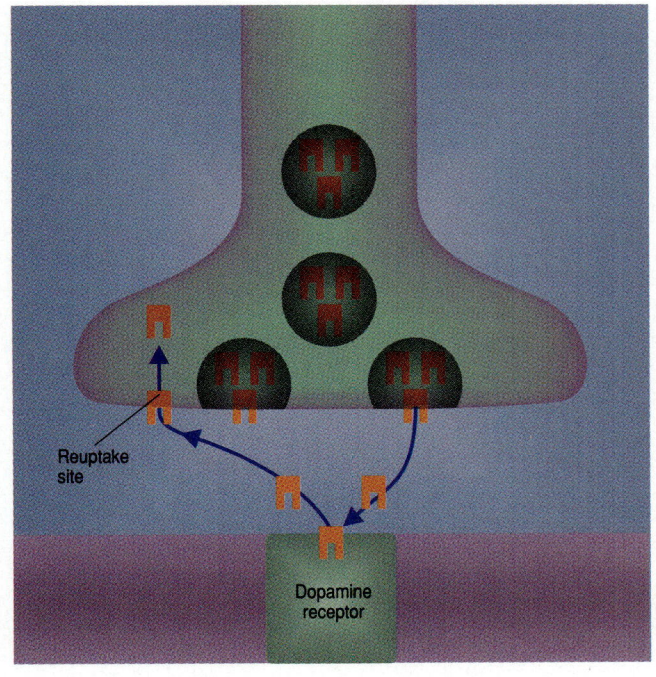

CHEMICAL (COCAINE)

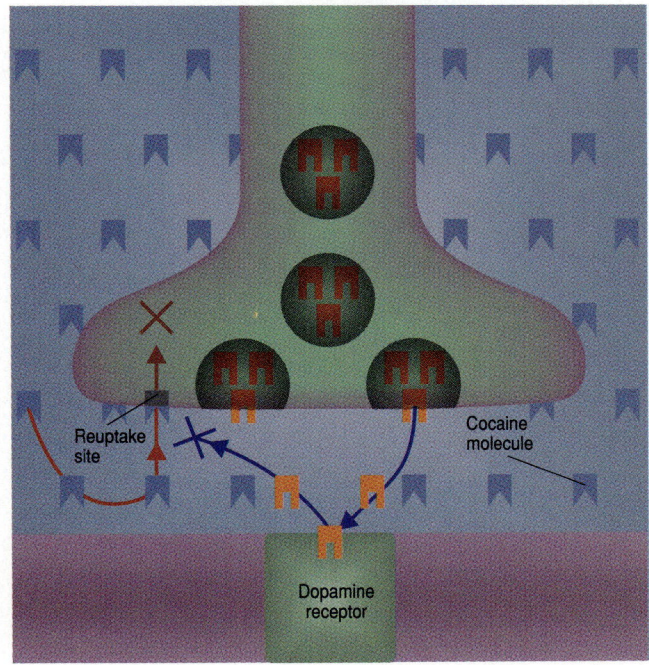

MECHANISMS OF DRUG BINDING

The successful neurotransmission of the natural opiate endorphin is shown at top left. The opiate drug morphine, though, floods the synapse, binds to and activates the receptor sites of the natural opiate as shown top right. In the case of cocaine, however, the drug binds to the reuptake site (bottom right) so that the natural neurotransmitter dopamine cannot reenter its home neuron after release. This then increases the amount of dopamine in the synapse.

The mechanism of alcohol intoxication is less understood. Taking a drink initially stimulates, then depresses brain function, including the systems that moderate feelings and behavior. Cares slip away, possibly because alcohol may affect the uptake of GABA. Other neurons may also be affected, including those for dopamine, noradrenaline, serotonin, acetylcholine and endorphins. One theory holds that alcohol works in the brain by disturbing the lipid membrane that is responsible for regulating the internal environment of brain cells.

Of the billions of people who add sparkle to their lives with a glass of wine or a sip of whiskey, a relatively large proportion—perhaps 5 percent—become alcoholics. Some drink heavily for the sheer thrill of getting drunk and are often prone to violence when inebriated. Others seem to take alcohol for its sedative value, as a kind of readily available tranquilizer. Both binge drinkers and steady heavy-use drinkers may do terrible damage to their brains. Long-term alcohol

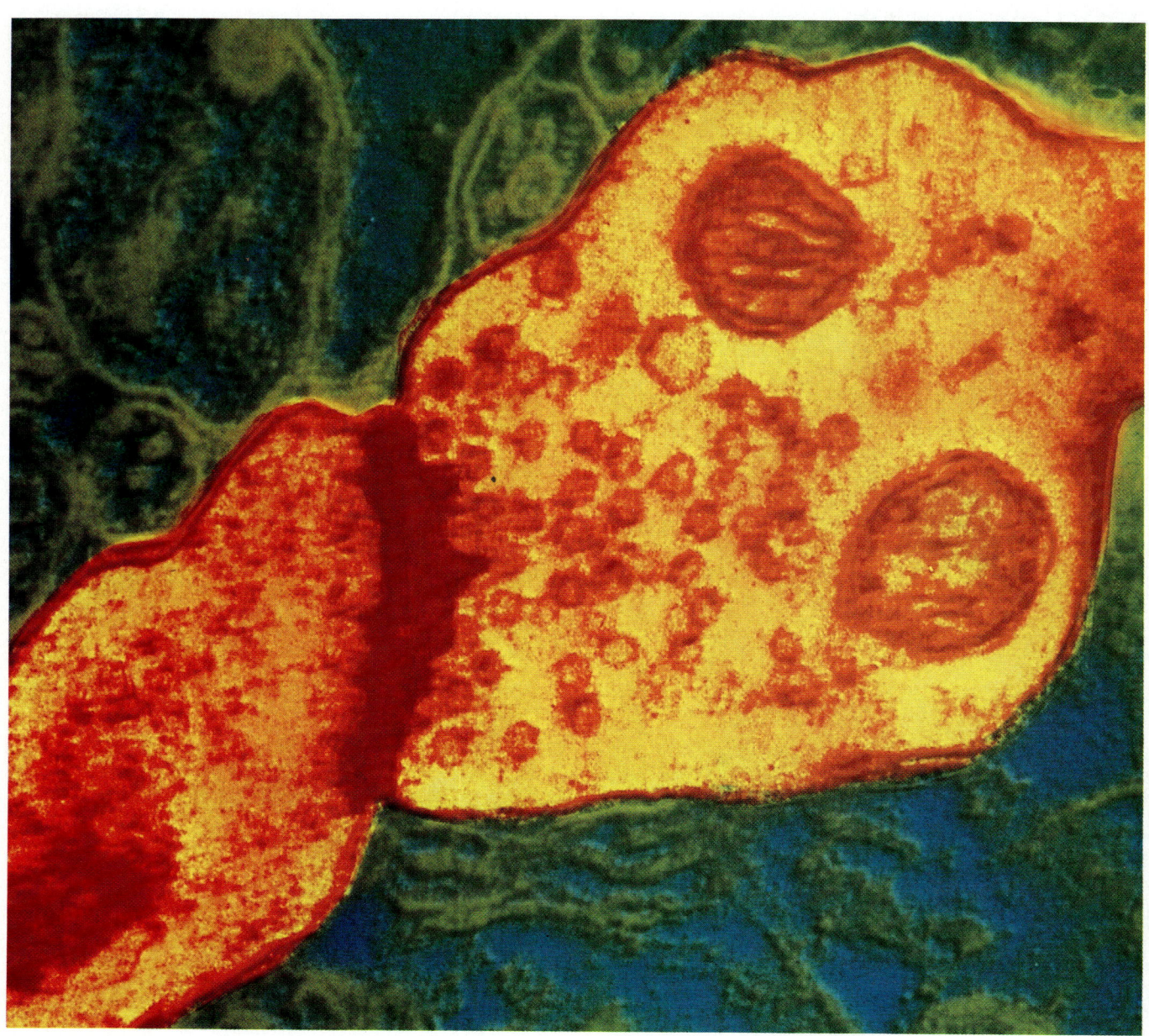

An artificially colored synapse is caught in action by microphotography. An electrical signal travels along the axon at left to trigger the release of neurotransmitter stored in the tiny red circular vesicles. The neurotransmitter moves into the gap, or synaptic cleft, here seen as a thick red band separating the end of the axon from the next yellow nerve cell at the right of the photograph. The neurotransmitter binds to a receptor on the second cell.

Drugs	Short-term effect	Long-term effect	Withdrawal symptoms
CNS STIMULANT (cocaine)	- local anesthesia; increased energy, alertness; sense of power	- destroyed nasal tissue (if sniffed); strong psychological dependence	- depression
CNS STIMULANT (amphetamines)	- reduced appetite; increased heart rate, blood pressure	- malnutrition; psychological dependence	- protracted sleep; depression; large appetite
RAPID-ACTING OPIATES (heroin, morphine, meperidine)	- pain relief; contentment; emotional detachment	- weight loss; reduced sex hormone levels; physical, psychological dependence	- cramps, gooseflesh, diarrhea
NICOTINE (tobacco, smoked)	- increased pulse rate, blood pressure; reduced appetite; relaxes regular users	- physical, psychological dependence; respiratory disease; certain cancer risks	————
MINOR TRANQUILIZERS (benzodiazepines)	- reduced emotional responses, alertness; muscle relaxant	- physical, psychological dependence	- anxiety; sleep disturbances
SEDATIVE HYPNOTICS (barbiturates)	- reduced tension; sleep; intoxication in high doses	- physical, psychological dependence; sleep disturbances	- anxiety; possible delirium tremens and convulsions
ALCOHOL	- reduced coordination; suppressed inhibitions; slow mental processes	- physical, psychological dependence; risk of brain, nerve, heart damage, cirrhosis, certain cancers	- delirium tremens; convulsions
CAFFEINE (coffee, tea, cocoa, some soft drinks)	- increased alertness, pulse rate	- mild physical dependence; stomach ulceration	- irritability; restlessness
CANNABIS (marijuana, hashish)	- euphoria	- loss of drive; impaired learning ability	————
HALLUCINOGENS (LSD, mescaline, MDMA)	- perceptual distortion; arousal	- flashbacks, possible brain damage	————

All of the above drugs, with the exception of cannabis and the hallucinogens are physically addictive, attributable exclusively to the pharmacological actions of the drugs on the `reward system' of the brain. The rank order of their addictiveness on the chart can be affected by social and economic factors or by personality differences in users.

DRUGS OF ABUSE

Among the most dangerous abused substances are those that are socially condoned. Opium and cocaine were once legally sanctioned, as the potentially deadly drugs nicotine and alcohol remain today. Social, personal and economic factors contribute to the drugs' intrinsic addictiveness, which is ranked on a decreasing scale on this chart.

abuse can destroy neurons in the brain leading to disorientation, impaired memory, depressed intellectual functioning, decreased judgment and even dementia. For chronic alcoholics, withdrawal—with delirium tremens and its convulsions and visions—may be fatal without treatment.

Not all drugs are physically addictive. The lure of marijuana and hashish seems to be primarily psychological. Psychedelics such as LSD and mescaline—which closely resemble the transmitters serotonin and noradrenaline in molecular structure—appear to ignite no physical or psychological dependency. Cocaine, though it creates a strong psychological dependency, spawns only mild physical dependency. But nicotine, in addition to all the black mischief smoking deposits in the lungs and arteries, is difficult to give up because it, too, is addictive. What is surprising is that even the so-called hard drugs such as cocaine and the opiates do not invariably result in a lifetime of drugged-out purgatory. Contrary to popular belief, on average only about 10 percent of the people who have ever snorted coke or shot up with heroin have gone on to become full-fledged addicts.

The reason some people get hooked while others do not remains one of the great enigmas of psychological research. Environment must certainly be a factor. Heredity seems to play a part; both alcoholism and other drug abuse tends to run in families. But no one is genetically predestined to become an alcoholic or a drug addict. Even if the genetic missing link were found, the interaction of all the external environmental factors can never be ignored. Human beings need satisfaction, stimulation and pleasure. If no healthy means to achieve these can be found, the choice can all too easily become chemical.

Natural Highs

It is mood altering and habit forming, but it's totally chemical free. Those who derive pleasure from climbing mountains without safety ropes, maneuvering a vehicle at life-endangering speeds, or free-falling from an aircraft at 3,500 feet are extreme examples of the human need for stimulation. Yet not all thrills are physical. Trailblazing scientists, high-stakes entrepreneurs—and even shoplifters—are different types of risktakers, seeking out novelty, conflict, challenge.

What motivates behaviors with such a range of health hazards, rewards and social acceptance is itself a risky question, open to the thrill-seeking psychologist. Low arousability of the reticular activating system, and over- or under-stimulation in the early months of life are possibilities under investigation.

The euphoria commonly known as "runner's high" is more than habit forming—it is pharmacologically addictive. Intense physical exertion causes the pituitary gland to increase production of endorphins and enkephalins, the brain's natural opiates, creating a morphine-like euphoria and dulling perception.

During a heavy exercise regime—jogging seven miles a day or more, for instance—an athlete's brain can become dependent on a high turnover of these mood-altering neurotransmitters. Athletes who abruptly cease training frequently experience mild opiate-withdrawal symptoms which might include irritability, muddled thinking and disrupted sleep.

An insatiable hunger for healthy physical activity must be, for the most part, a benign addiction. The good news for thrill-seekers is that the world needs these restless souls as much as they, themselves, need stimulation. Through the ages, human progress has depended on individuals ready to go out on a limb to promote ideas that have seemed downright outlandish. Could it be that the contributions of a Columbus or a Galileo were made for the thrill of it all?

Individuals with thrill-seeking personalities may have brains that require high-octane stimulation to get revved up. For some, the insecurity of mountain climbing causes a pleasurable rush of elation.

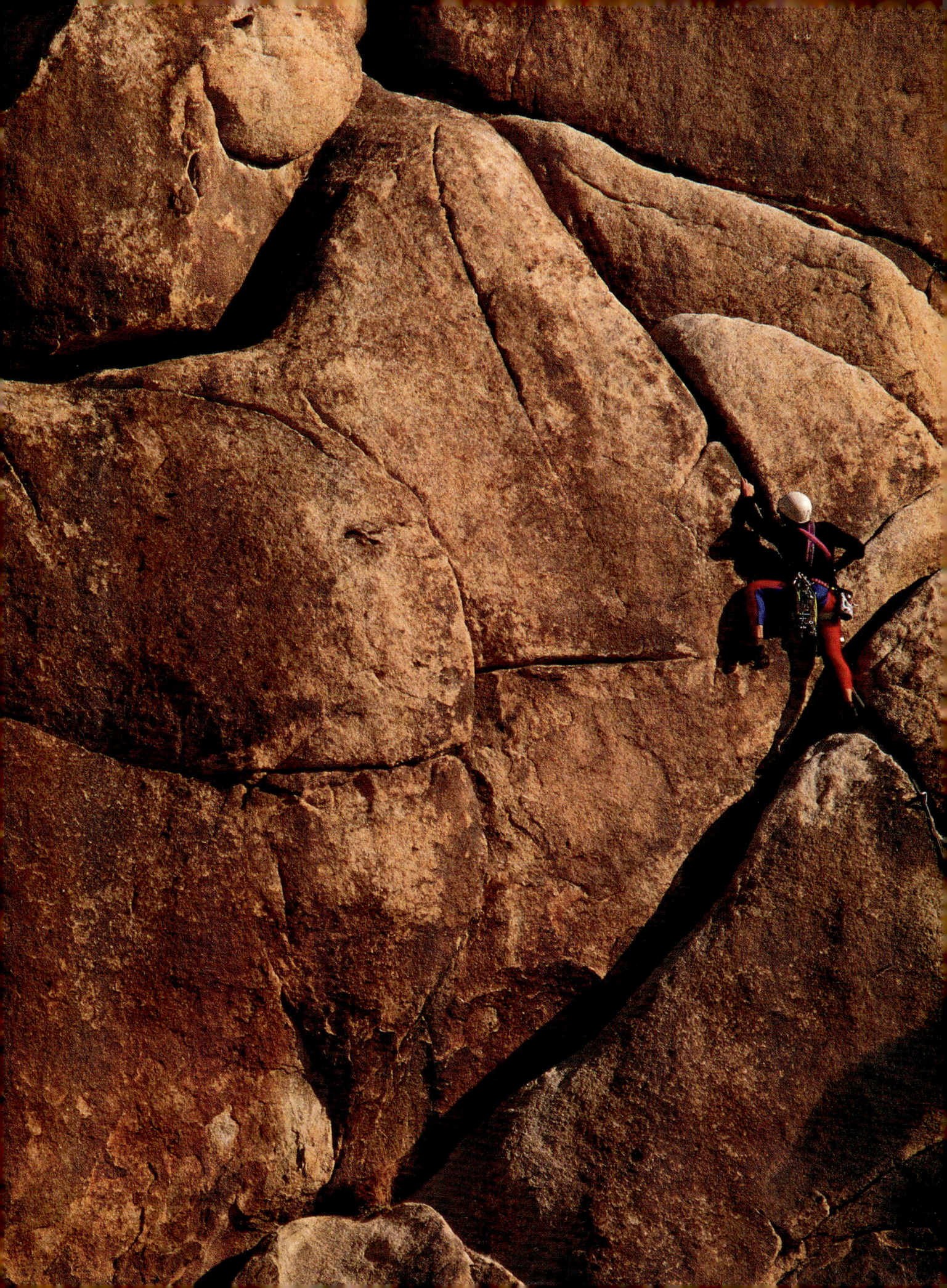

NETWORKS OF BRILLIANCE

Gathered in folds like a silk scarf in a magician's hand, the capacious surface of the cerebral cortex appears deceptively unassuming. Yet within the rounded hills and steep valleys of the human cortex operates the most highly evolved colossus of electrical engineering known, networks of neurons in a constant buzz of communication. It is fitting that the crowning glory of the human machine should take the loftiest position, not only atop the body, but over the team of parts comprising the brain itself. The cortex is the seat of the highest functions of which the human race is capable, distinguishing humans from all other animals and making possible their most brilliant achievements.

Beings as simple as mollusks learn and remember, and use learned material to their advantage. It may be that human memory shares biochemical similarities with this distant relative, but a quick comparison of scale is staggering. Whereas the nervous system of the sea snail *Aplysia*—the focus of current learning and memory studies—contains about 10,000 neurons, the human cortex contains more than a million times that.

The truly great feats of the human brain are communication and abstract thinking. The study of people who exhibited speech problems after sustaining head injuries led to the theory that linguistic activity was localized, in most individuals, in the left cerebral hemisphere. Scientists have since mapped the principal regions involved in decoding spoken or written language, planning verbal speech and the very act of thinking itself.

In an era of increasing reliance on thinking machines, fruits of the human imagination whose prowess some see as threatening the raison d'être of their creators, it is comforting to know that the human intellect is vastly superior in many respects to even the most complex computer. The computer is a logic machine that runs on programs whose steps are arranged one after the other in a single chain. The brain does not work in such a neat—and limited—fashion, but "in parallel." Intu-

---

Neurons, wired into dense networks of cellular switches, produce a synaptic synergy that defies measurement. Even the most sophisticated computer hardware cannot rival the "wetware" of the human brain.

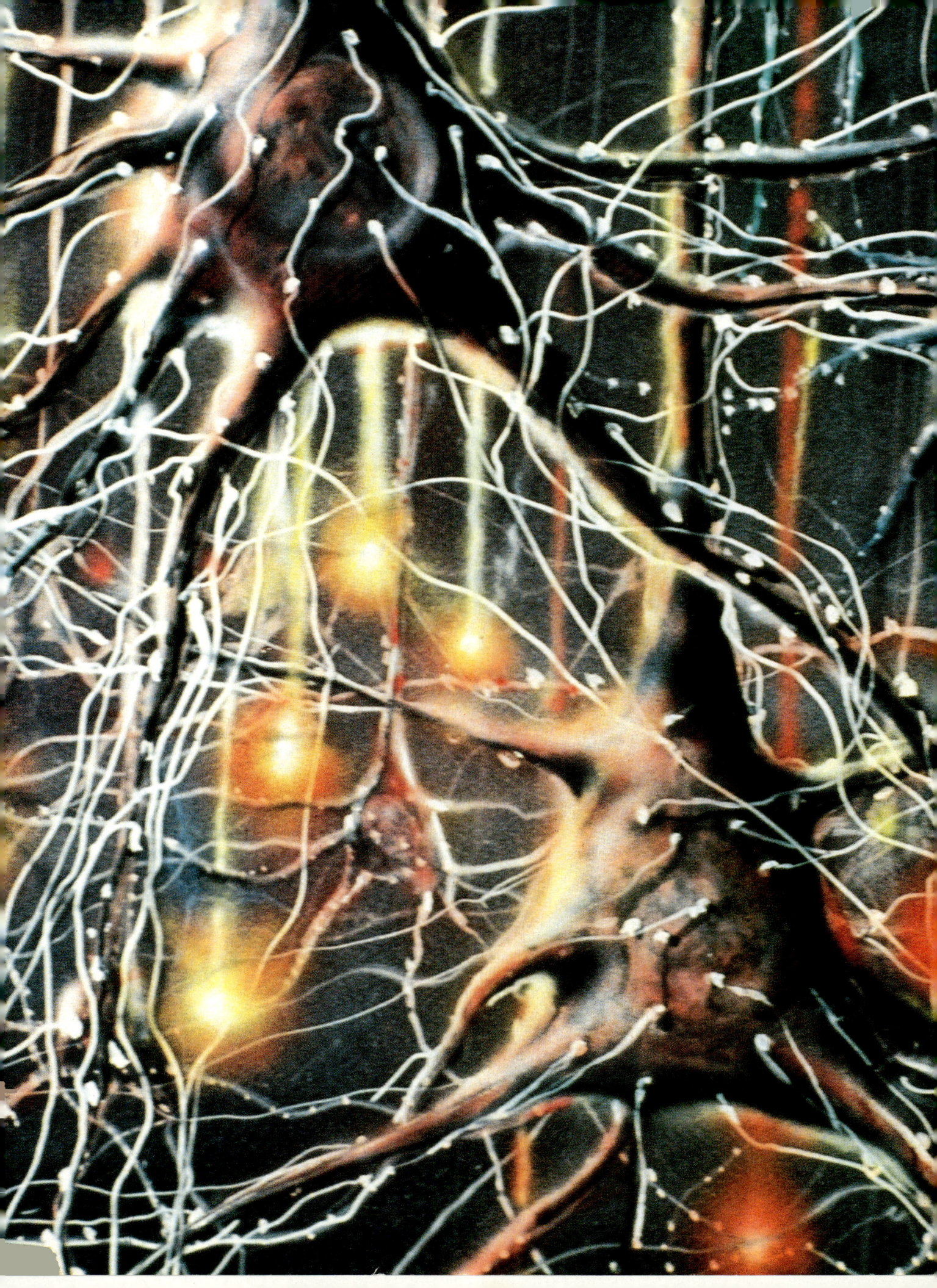

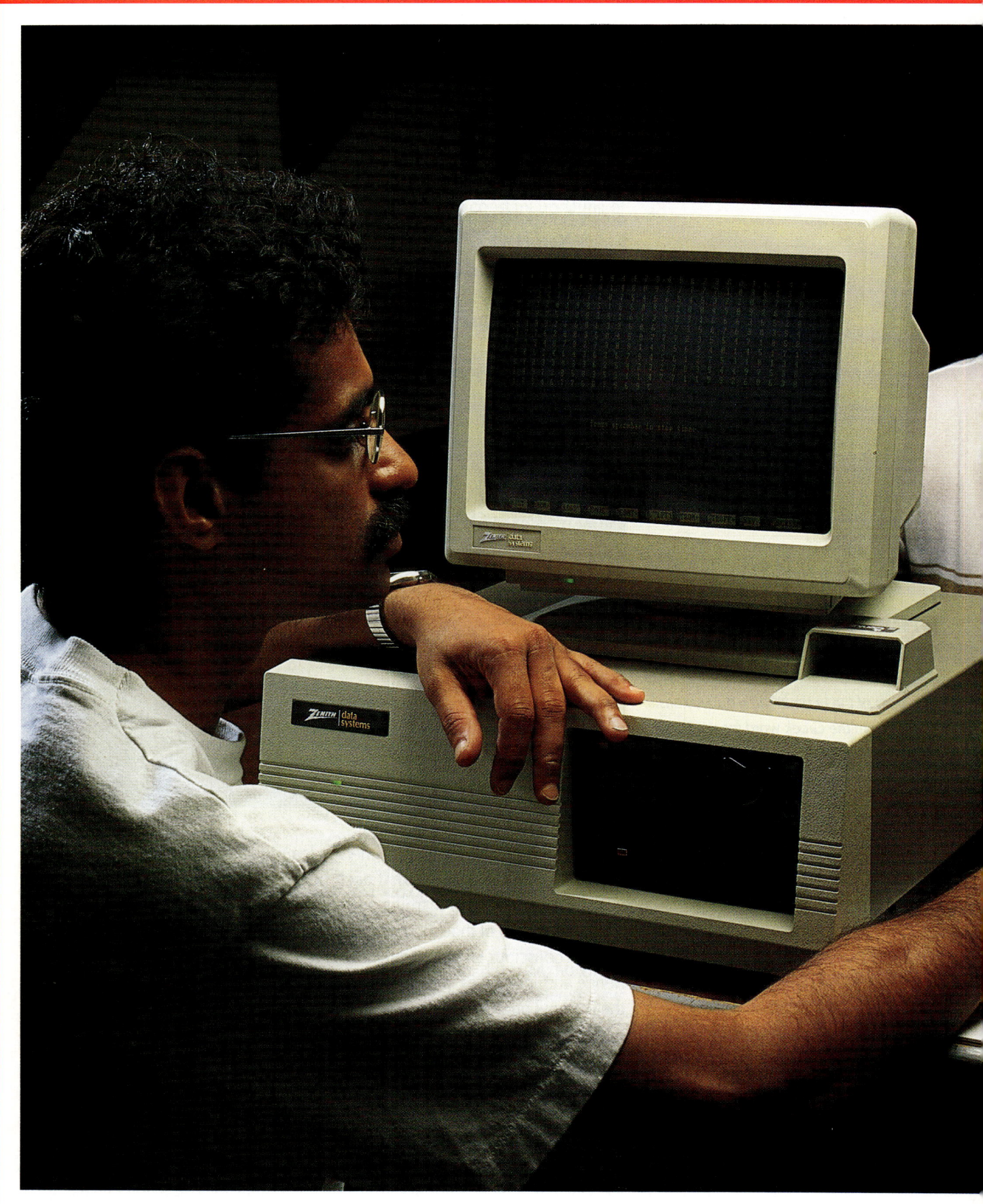

110

NETWORKS OF BRILLIANCE

Rajan the Pi-Man

His first memory: MYX1689, a license plate. He was three years old. Most people can remember the seven digits of a phone number long enough to dial or jot it down. Some can handle a long-distance number and area code—10 digits—while a rare few manage a credit card number. Then there is Rajan Mahadevan, whose number-crunching memory could recall all the winning numbers in a lottery draw, after hearing them only once.

Rajan is devoted to learning the first 100,000 digits of pi, the ratio of a circle's circumference to its diameter. Math teachers are often content with the three-digit version: 3.14. Rajan, however, has already publicly recited as far as the 31,811th digit—he got stuck on the 31,812th digit, 5.

At Kansas State University, where Rajan is both a student and the subject of a memory study, scientists are studying the brain behind the memory. Though the way his memory works is still a mystery, tests pitting Rajan against control subjects reveal idiosyncrasies in his way of encoding information. For example, while he surpasses others in memorizing lists of unrelated words, surprisingly he falls behind with words that share common themes. The reason? Whereas most people have better recall for words they can group—types of trees, cities, colors—to Rajan's rote mind they are all perceived as equal data, like numbers.

The aesthetic experience of a melodious string of digits makes his "hair stand on end," but unlike the famous Russian memorist "S," whose recollections of individual digits were peopled with fat women and crippled men, no such vivid imagery colors Rajan's abstract mind. A geometric figure described by a control subject as a "caved-in barn," might receive from Rajan a highly mathematical epithet, such as "trapezium."

KSU investigators have proved that memory improves with practice, but Rajan believes that genetic factors contribute to his brain's strong predisposition. While his father at one point knew every line of all 154 Shakespearean sonnets by heart, his maternal grandfather, like Rajan, had a natural talent for numbers.

Though Rajan says he doesn't rely on mnemonic devices, certain digit clusters echo trivia facts in his head. For example, the digits 1745 are filed away by Rajan as 39. Why? Because he remembers that Benjamin Franklin was born in 1706 and thus would have been 39 in 1745.

Easy as pi!

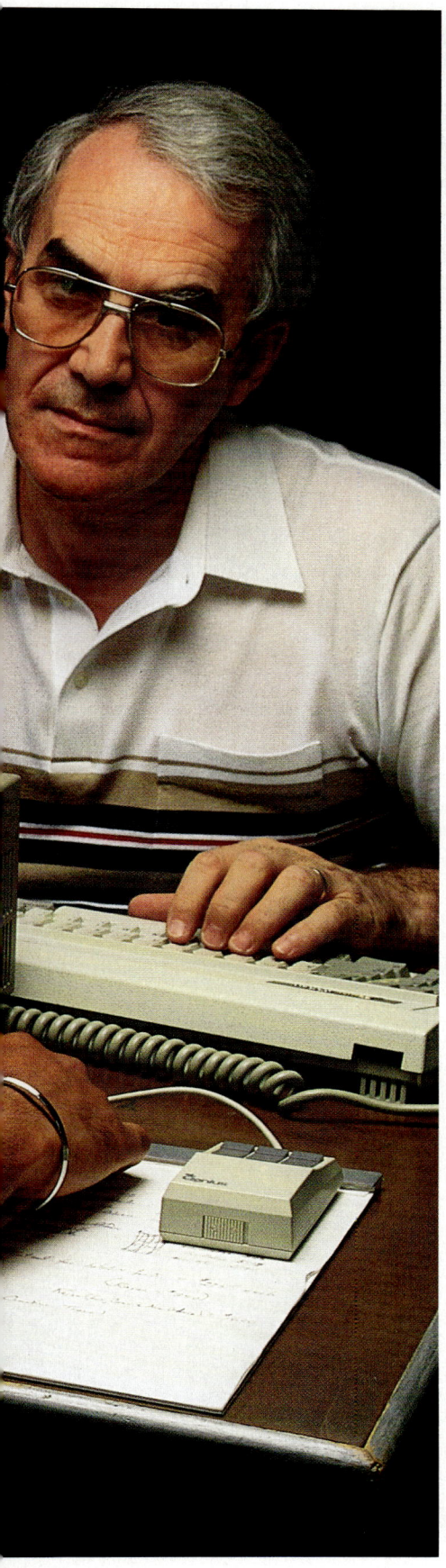

Rajan Mahadevan works regularly with Dr. Charles Thompson, a professor of psychology at Kansas State University in Manhattan, Kansas. Given a series of five numbers from anywhere in the first 10,000 digits of pi, Rajan can go on and list the next five.

information, proceeds to short-term storage and then culminates in more-or-less permanent storage. The first step along the route to knowledge is iconic memory. For a second or so, anything a person sees is retained in a near-perfect photographic image. If, for instance, a card with a telephone number is flashed before a person's eyes and then turned over, he or she can still "read" it correctly from iconic memory. Scientists believe that transient photochemical changes in the eye's retina are responsible for a continuous, movie-like stream of such fast-decaying images.

This input, like impressions from the other senses, is routed to the cortex along neural pathways that hone raw data into complex perceptions. Without rehearsal, these perceptions may remain in short-term memory for a few minutes at most. This process is believed to take place in the inferior temporal cortex and the hippocampus. Short-term memory mediates contact with the here-and-now, furnishing a person's moment-to-moment consciousness with new perceptions. Because it is the interface between consciousness and current experience, short-term memory is also called working memory.

The storage capacity of short-term memory is very limited, however. Test subjects given a quick look at lists of items such as numbers, colors and words and then asked to recall them, on average can remember seven. In addition to individual bits of information such as single digits or letters, the "magic number seven" includes, as single items, multiple-bit "chunks"—words, simple geometric figures, the notes of a musical phrase. Bundling information into chunks allows short-term memory to handle more data simultaneously. The seven digits of the number 1000000 fill the average short-term memory to capacity, but there is room to spare if it is converted to three chunks—1,000,000.

Techniques such as chunking and repetition help the mind hold material, but other processes, some of them beyond conscious control, also help determine which perceptions and thoughts are plucked from the stream continuously rushing through short-term memory for transfer to long-term memory. Emotions, for instance, influence the selection of material for storage. Monkeys, normally fast learners when rewarded, have difficulty remembering that successful performance of a task results in the pleasure of a reward if they have had the amygdala removed. This structure is a vital part of the mood-related limbic system. Nerve fibers carrying data from all of the sensory systems in the cortex converge on the same part of the amygdala. This circuit also sends axons to the hypothalamus, which neuroscientists believe plays a strong role in forming emotional responses.

Removing the amygdala may wipe away the emotional coloration of stimuli and deprive the animal of what may be the single most important means of evaluating their significance for survival. Emotions, then, might act as the filter for the perceptual flood, directing the mind to snatch out meaningful information and let the rest go by. Because it is interposed between the senses and the emotions, the amygdala may play a pivotal role in selecting memories for long-term storage.

As closely linked as short-term and long-term memory are, they are very different phenomena. Short-term memory is dynamic and evanescent, while long-term memory involves permanent neurochemical change that can result in memories lasting a lifetime. Strong evidence of two separate phenomena came from surgical patients like H.M. as well as from victims of still more drastic disorders of the limbic system. Korsakov's syndrome, a result of chronic alcoholism, can

THE UNCORRUGATED CORTEX
As the human brain evolved, ingenious nature tucked the expanding cortex into intricate folds so that it could be contained inside the skull. The tremendous volume of the cortex makes possible an astronomical combination of neural networks. Unfolded it would necessitate a hugely disproportionate head.

erase entire decades from memory and block the storage of any new long-term memories while leaving short-term memory amazingly intact. The active process of memory storage involves the temporal lobe and the hippocampus, but long-term memory does not appear to be limited to a particular site. Neurobiologists have not determined where memories are stored or how they are recalled, but the functions appear to be widely distributed in the human brain.

Dr. Eric Kandel and his colleagues at Columbia University in New York have spent years studying the primitive learning and memory processes of *Aplysia*, the marine snail with an unusually accessible nervous system containing only 10,000 or so neurons, all of them conveniently large. One revealing behavior is the gill withdrawal reflex or the snail's reaction when a jet of water is squirted to some part of its body. Initially the snail withdraws the gill protectively, but after a training session of 10 squirts the reaction is much reduced. This change in behavior, which reflects a type of learning called habituation, may remain for several weeks. Habituation has high survival value, since it allows animals to focus on important stimuli rather than wasting attention on the insignificant.

With glass microelectrodes Kandel has identified the individual cells controlling gill action. The sensory cells that are stimulated by the water jet fire impulses to a group of motor cells, which in turn synapse with muscle cells in the gills. An examination of the synapses between sensory and motor cells in habituated snails shows that the quantity of neurotransmitter released by the sensory cells is reduced as is the activation of the motor neurons. When the training sessions are repeated for a few days, the reduction in neurotransmitter output can persist for three weeks—which, in snails, constitutes long-term memory. The opposite of habituation is the learning process called sensitization. With sensitization, repeated stimulus causes an increase rather than a decrease in response—either because the stimulus is noxious or because of the characteristics of the particular neurons.

Sensitization results in actual structural changes to dendrites, which can be detected by electron microscopes. This led Kandel and his colleagues to think that the functional and structural changes account for both short-term and long-term memory in *Aplysia*. Learning, it appears, can take place in a very simple neural pathway that has at least one function—in this case, gill withdrawal—while in the brains of more complex animals, neural pathways might be able to store many different memories and accommodate a multitude of other functions as well.

It is uncertain whether the neural mechanisms underlying habituation in higher animals are essentially identical with those in simple systems such as that of *Aplysia*, but this type of learning is virtually universal. Human infants learn by habituation almost from birth. A baby only four hours old will stop sucking to listen intently to an unfamiliar tone. After several repetitions it ignores the tone and goes back to sucking, once again stopping to listen if a new tone is sounded.

Learning to associate two stimuli that occur simultaneously is a more complex task. Called classical conditioning, the process was discovered by Russian physiologist Ivan Pavlov. He noticed that when the dogs he used in experiments were hungry, they salivated at the sight of their empty food dish, just as they did when they saw food. Classical conditioning links a stimulus that naturally prompts a particular response with an originally neutral stimulus—for Pavlov's dogs, food and a dish. Timing is a critical element. If the two are presented closely in time, the neutral stimulus becomes so strongly associated with the potent one that it eventually evokes exactly the same reaction in the subject—in this case, salivation.

Classical conditioning is equally effective when the unconditioned stimulus provokes fear or pain. Dr. Daniel L. Alkon of the National Institute of Neurological and Communicative Disorders and Stroke in Maryland taught a marine snail, *Hermissenda*, to associate a flash of light with turbulent water. Either stimulus then prompted the snail to tighten its hold on a firm surface—a move that prevents its being swept away. Alkon and his group have found that several chemical and structural changes appeared in the conditioned snails.

Neuronal circuits in the brains of conditioned rabbits have been found to change structurally and biochemically, like those of *Hermissenda*. Such evidence prompted Alkon to hypothesize that what an animal learns is stored as a uniquely patterned set of changes concentrated in synapses. Although they are no longer capable of dividing in mature animals, neurons can nevertheless undergo remarkable dendritic transformations that capture experience and store it for days, weeks or even longer. In higher animals, huge numbers of neurons may transform themselves and establish connections to form an assembly holding a durable memory. The original sensory event—or one very like it—can trigger electrical signals that reactivate the assembly and the memory it holds.

Habituation, sensitization and classical conditioning confer procedural knowledge. How much overlap there is between the neural mechanisms of these noncognitive learning processes and those that channel declarative knowledge into human memory is simply unknown. Moreover, progress toward a definitive answer may be frustratingly slow, especially if it can come only from a study of

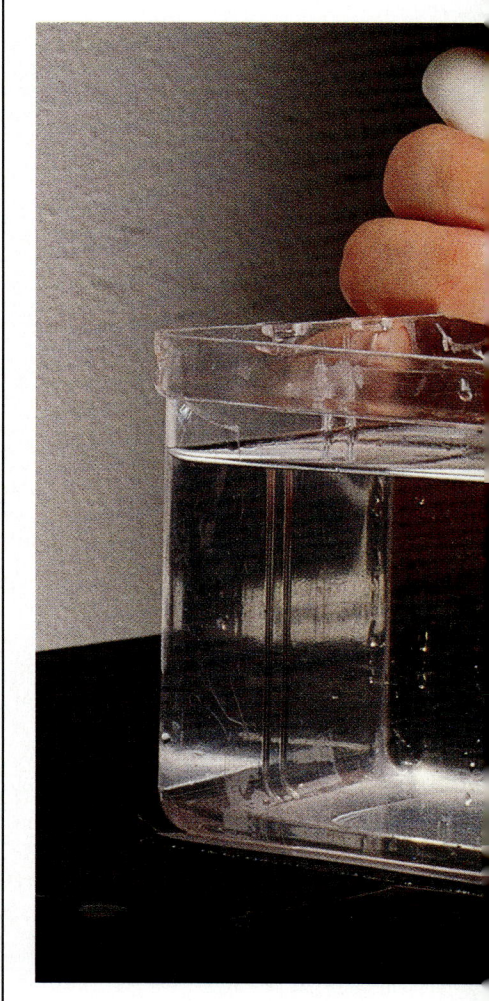

the human brain. Obviously, only a very narrow range of experiments is possible with people, and even a thorough understanding of learning and memory in as close a relative of humans as the chimpanzee can leave critical gaps. Ninety-nine percent of our genetic material is shared with chimpanzees, the most intelligent of the apes, but the other one percent seems to have changed so radically since evolutionary paths diverged 25 million years ago that humans have made a qualitative leap forward in brain architecture and function.

BEYOND THE HERE AND NOW

Language is the behavior that most definitively divides human from ape. No other species has anything approaching this system of representation that allows its members to communicate thought and emotion and to encode information for storage and cognition. Animals communicate effectively with their kind, but their utterances are typically stereotyped and rigidly determined. Language, on the other hand, is so flexible that it allows people to generate sentences that are unique, yet instantly understandable by other speakers of the same language. Primatologist Jane Goodall has remarked, "Language enables us to make meaningful plans not only for the immediate future, which even the chimp can do, but for the next year

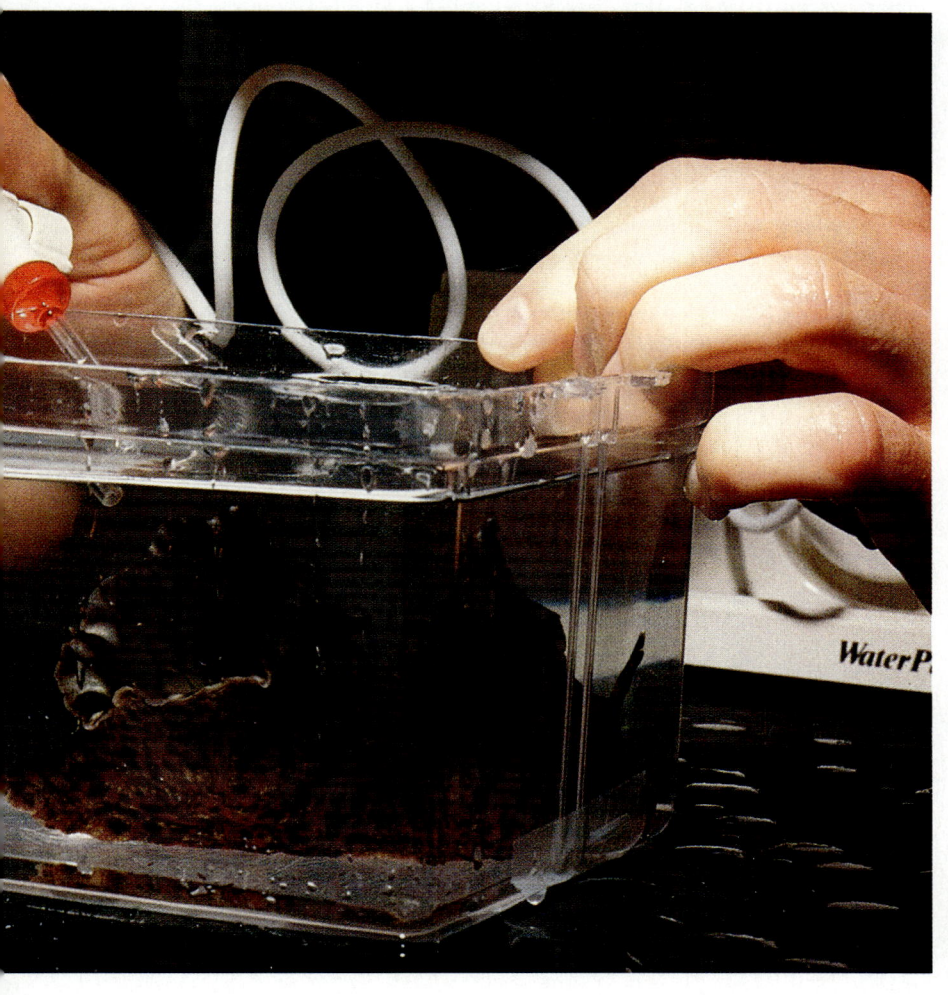

MOLLUSK MEMORIES

Neurochemical research would crawl at a snail's pace if not for invertebrate models such as *Aplysia*. The neurons of invertebrates are not only few in number, but also are organized with remarkable similarity between members of the species—something not true in humans, even in identical twins. *Aplysia* has the added advantage of having big, easy-to-spot neurons, many of which can be viewed by the naked eye.

Neuroscientists recognize that invertebrate studies give a limited picture of how human brain cells work. Yet although they are by no means identical, human and snail neurons share fundamental structural and chemical properties. *Aplysia* uses some of the same neurotransmitters found in the human brain, and scientists believe that similar synaptic mechanisms will show them how both people and snails learn and remember.

Irritating the sea snail's gill with a squirt of water provokes a reflex mediated by neurotransmission at specific synapses. Lab experiments such as this are shedding light on the workings of the human brain.

The Agony of Alzheimer's

PET scans, used to trace the sad progress of AD, reveal the decrease in metabolic activity. The lights dim, then go out.

Under the microscope, AD's signature is unveiled. Neurofibrillary tangles—pairs of fine, twisted nerve fibers—cut a swath inside healthy cells (arrow above left). *What is left behind are neuritic plaques, or "tombstones," degenerating bits of nerve cells surrounding a core of fibrous material called amyloid* (arrow directly below).

For scientists prying open the Pandora's box that is Alzheimer's disease, the task is almost as overwhelming as is remembering the way home for a victim of the disorienting dementia. Unleashed are complex puzzles of cognitive and behavioral abnormalities, gross and microscopic anatomical damage, and neurochemical and genetic aberrations.

An estimated 10 percent of those over 65 show symptoms of Alzheimer's—first memory loss, then erosion of other mental and physical functions. With so much at stake in a rapidly aging population, the race is on to conquer the degenerative and irreversible disease that kills twice —first the brain, then the body.

Researchers now have a scale, called FAST (functional assessment stages), by which to measure precisely the onset and course of AD. Virtually every victim follows the same sequence, losing cognitive and motor abilities in the exact reverse order and in roughly the same amount of time that they were gained in the formative years. In a cruel irony of nature, the devastating course of AD is the mirror image of human development.

Even a cursory reading of the list of possible causes—genetic, toxic, viral, neurochemical, immunological—suggests that interconnection is involved. Some trigger, perhaps environmental, begins the chain reaction of devastation.

Is it possible to intervene?

With every refinement in measuring brain neurochemicals comes the possibility for new drug therapies. Clinical trials are under way for drugs that inhibit an enzyme that breaks down acetylcholine, a neurotransmitter associated with memory. In other promising research, an organic chemical called nerve growth factor (NGF), which nourishes and recharges nerve cells, is being infused into damaged cells in rats. The cells survive. Neural cell implants, to replace dead cells, are also being tested. Genetic research has focused on chromosome 21 as a possible location of an abnormal gene responsible for AD. Victims of Down's syndrome, who also suffer premature aging and AD-type symptoms, have an extra chromosome 21. Investigation continues into genes on this and other chromosomes.

For many of the possible drug therapies, a way must be found to bypass the blood-brain barrier, which blocks most chemicals. Drug, cell and NGF implants are still experimental surgical procedures with consequent risks. But in research labs around the world, both optimism and progress are taking quantum leaps.

In autopsy, brains of AD patients reveal a characteristic pattern of tissue and weight loss. Where a normal brain (in cross section, left) may weigh up to 1,400 grams, an AD brain (right) may weigh 500 grams less. Striking tissue loss is seen in the major convolutions along the surface, the temporal lobes and near the ventricles, the central cavities that carry cerebrospinal fluid.

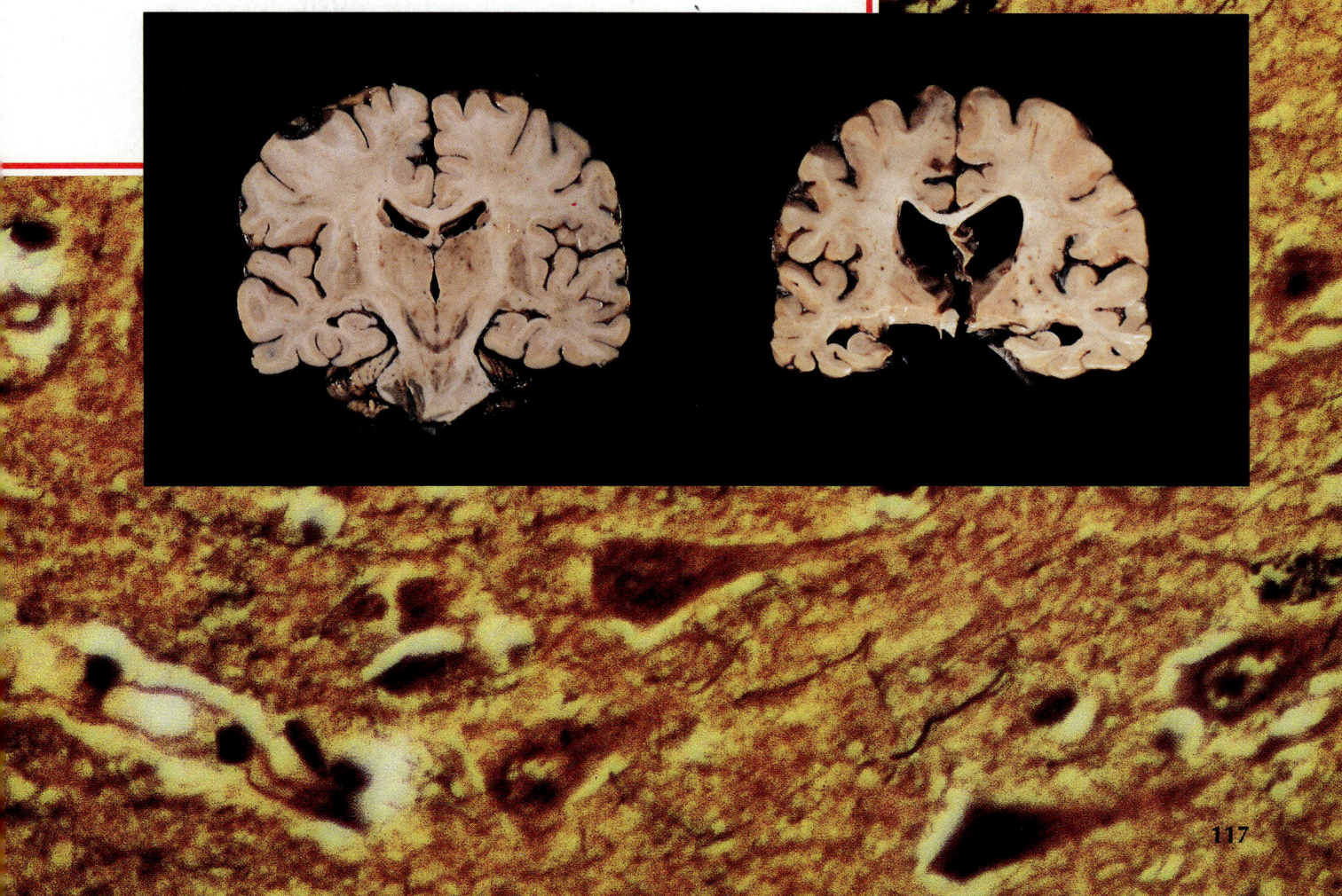

or 10 years ahead. It enables us to pass on traditions and cultures to our children about types of behavior or objects that are not present. We can talk about them, we can explain them, and in this way we are completely and utterly different from the chimpanzees."

Well before their first birthday, all normal children living in an ordinary social setting, no matter what their culture, are receptive to the sounds and vocabulary, the grammar and syntax of their native language. Children born deaf show the same spontaneous urge to communicate. If parents use sign language, their child will begin to sign at about six months of age. Although acquiring language involves learning, there is a great deal of evidence that it is an innate, genetically determined biological process with universal and predictable stages. Like kittens, monkeys and other mammalian newborns, babies are instinctively attuned to sounds critical to their survival, cooing and gesturing in response to the human voice. At six months or so, a child recognizes and categorizes vowels and consonants. In another six months they are used in single words. By two the child has begun to master grammar, the rules governing combinations of words. Depending on the language the child learns, the elements of grammar may include word order along with concepts such as number, agency, reciprocity, gender and time. A 1,000-word vocabulary and a solid grasp of grammar are characteristic of the three-year-old. Entire sentences now come easily to the child because of a growing familiarity with syntax, which supplies the patterns for combining grammatical units into meaningful messages. Oddly enough, sexual maturation has a significant effect on language behavior. The physical changes responsible have not been identified, but it is far more difficult to learn a new language after puberty.

According to the widely accepted theory of psycholinguist Noam Chomsky of the Massachusetts Institute of Technology, every child is born with an innate, genetically determined knowledge of a universal set of grammatical rules. This grammar allows children to infer from the conversation of family and friends the parameters governing their particular native language. At the same time, they learn the characteristics of its sound system. From the hundreds of distinct sounds the human voice can produce, for instance, English uses at least 36 phonemes, or meaningfully different sounds. Each language makes its own arbitrary selection, and infants quickly attune to sounds weighted with meaning.

Language is the only such complex system humans conquer so readily and without formal instruction. There is no evidence that correcting a young child's errors is helpful, and a parent who habitually points out mistakes may actually be an impediment. Children need no more help learning their language than they do learning to walk.

How the brain processes auditory intake and produces oral output has been a target for neuroscientists since the mid-19th Century. Virtually from the outset,

THE DIVIDED BRAIN
The hemispheres of the cerebral cortex share more similarities than differences. In most people, the left hemisphere handles all types of language—the sole unilateral function. The right hemisphere is more

the investigation of language has been coupled with the broader phenomenon of laterality—the division of cognitive labor between the left and right hemispheres of the cerebral cortex. In 1861, French surgeon Pierre Paul Broca published the results of the autopsy he had performed on a longtime patient who had suffered from an aphasia, or language disorder. Although the man could understand language perfectly well, he had lost the ability to express his thoughts orally or in writing—the only word he could utter intelligibly was "tan." Broca found a small defect, or lesion, in the man's left frontal lobe. Over the next three years, Broca discovered similar lesions in eight more aphasic patients. Not all were so bereft of speech, but they shared a deterioration of grammar that limited their speech mainly to nouns and infinitives. The evidence from their autopsies prompted Broca to declare in his report, "Nous parlons avec l'hémisphère gauche!"

The startling implication that the brain is not functionally symmetrical was soon reinforced by German neurologist Karl Wernicke. He cared for several aphasics whose speech remained very fluent and structured, yet lacked appropriate nouns. Unlike Broca's patients, Wernicke's had lost not their powers of expression but their powers of comprehension. All the autopsies he performed revealed lesions in a specific area of the left hemisphere's temporal lobe.

The precise links he and Broca had discovered between aphasias and brain anatomy prompted Wernicke to postulate that language is processed serially in different regions, some of which are devoted to sensory components and some to motor components. In the aphasics he had examined, the lesion in what is now called Wernicke's area apparently disrupted visual and auditory perceptions of language so severely that the aphasic could no longer recognize them. Without recognition, comprehension was impossible. Reasoning that yet another distinct area must normally convey signals from the recognition area to the articulation area to complete the communication loop, Wernicke predicted that a lesion of this anatomical bridge would produce a "conduction aphasia." His prediction proved accurate. When the arcuate fasciculus, a bundle of fibers linking Broca's and Wernicke's areas, is diseased, the resulting aphasia prevents the patient from articulating phrases or even single words that he or she has just read or heard, despite normal comprehension. Lesions at other sites in the left hemisphere have equally devastating effects on language processes. Alexia—a total inability to read—results when a visual-input processing center near the boundary of the occipital and temporal lobes is diseased.

The left-right organization of the cerebral cortex has an interesting twist. Sensory and motor circuits tie each hemisphere to the contralateral, or opposite, side of the body. Sensory data received on one side of the body routinely cross over to the other side at several levels, including the spinal cord, the brainstem and the

efficient at visuo-spatial tasks such as facial and pattern recognition, as well as navigating in three-dimensional space. The bridge between the hemispheres, the corpus callosum, is the vital communication link.

brain itself, to register in the hemisphere on the opposite side. The preference for one hand over another reflects this neural organization. The differential functioning of eye and ear are not so noticeable, but right-handed people instinctively pay more attention to what appears in the right half of their visual field. An ingenious dichotic-listening test shows how finely attuned each ear is to the activities of the contralateral hemisphere. When a right-handed subject listens through headphones to different sets of digits, one played to the left ear and one to the right, he or she usually remembers more of the information picked up by the right ear. It has a distinct functional advantage over the left ear, since it delivers its data directly to the left hemisphere, which dominates verbal activity.

Events in the verbally dominant hemisphere can be tracked visually by PET scans. An injection of a harmless, short-lived radioactive isotope of oxygen is carried by the bloodstream to the brain. Picked up by the scanner and converted by computer into colored images, the energy emitted by the oxygen atoms shows changes in blood flow, which is greatest in areas where neurons are active. A group of Washington University Medical School researchers discovered that when a right-handed person reads a noun, blood flow in five different areas of the left occipital lobe increases. Only visual input has this impact. When the same noun is said aloud, it fails to trigger activity in these areas.

Neural networks for spoken language and for written language are left-hemisphere phenomena for well over 90 percent of right-handed people. One percent of righthanders are bilateral, calling both hemispheres into play for these tasks, and the remainder shift the function to the right hemisphere. Most left-handed people show the same pattern, but roughly a fifth of them favor the right hemisphere over the left, and more than 10 percent are bilateral.

Determining which hemisphere dominates linguistic processes is a simple but dramatic procedure. When the drug sodium amytal is injected into the left carotid artery, it quickly reaches the left hemisphere and suppresses its activity for several minutes. A temporary loss of speech points to the left hemisphere's dominance in that function. If injections to neither the right nor the left hemisphere suppress speech completely, the person is bilateral.

Although one hemisphere takes charge linguistically, the other—most frequently the right—has a critical complementary role. Every known language has musical qualities such as intonation, timing and volume that convey emotions profoundly affecting the meaning of a statement, sometimes contradicting its literal content altogether. The dichotic-listening test also demonstrates the right hemisphere's sensitivity to musical components. When a right-handed subject listens to two melodies simultaneously, he or she remembers better the one that is played to the left ear. The sites devoted to music are also thought by some to be involved in the emotional coloration of speech. These areas seem to be vulnerable to aprosodias—disorders in which speech sounds flat and monotonous.

What functional advantage lateralization offers is uncertain, but greater efficiency is one theoretical possibility. There is no doubt, however, that neural asymmetry has a long evolutionary pedigree. Even the 500,000-year-old Peking Man's skull bears the mark of a slightly larger left hemisphere. In modern humans

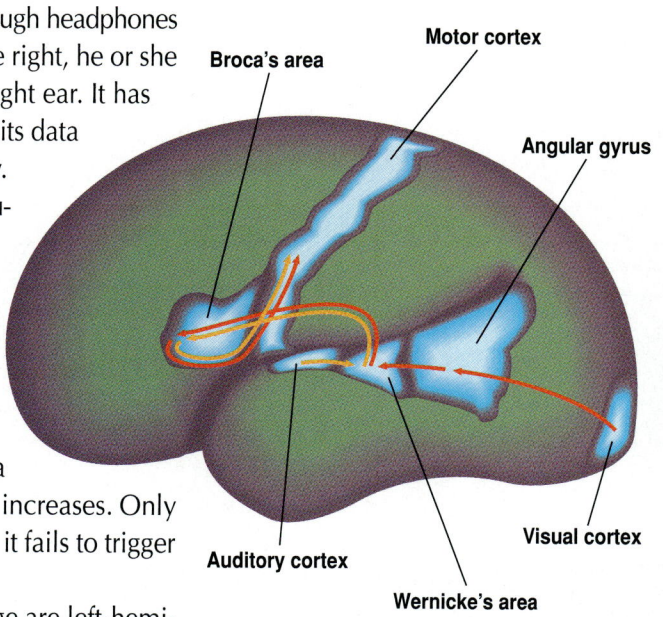

PATHWAYS OF LANGUAGE

While neurons in Wernicke's area are responsible for linguistic comprehension, those in Broca's area work with the motor cortex to produce speech. The red arrows trace the path followed when written words are read aloud. Words are detected by the eyes, sent to the visual cortex to be analyzed as visual patterns and then travel to an area called the angular gyrus, which associates the visual form of the word with the corresponding auditory pattern in Wernicke's area. From there the signals go to Broca's area and the section of the motor cortex that controls the mouth and tongue movements of speech. The yellow arrows show the path for repeating something heard. Nerve impulses go from the ear to the auditory cortex, but the words cannot be understood until the signals go to Wernicke's area. Since the words are to be spoken, the signals then go to Broca's area and the motor cortex for articulation.

with left-hemisphere dominance, a section of the temporal lobe where speech is processed is substantially larger than the corresponding part of the right hemisphere. The difference is already noticeable in a fetus at five months. Not surprisingly, the right hemisphere has its own characteristic enlargement—in the occipital lobe, which processes visual data.

Although the pattern of dominance takes shape before birth, a child's brain is plastic for several years. If the language-dominant hemisphere suffers damage, linguistic functions can shift to the other hemisphere. An extraordinary instance of plasticity occurs in deaf children who use sign language. Perceiving and analyzing movement is ordinarily the business of the right hemisphere, but the movements of sign language begin to be processed by the left hemisphere as the child learns to sign. The inborn language system apparently treats movement and sound as equivalents for expression.

While the two hemispheres have their own specializations, neurobiologists such as Brenda Milner caution against overemphasizing their differences at the expense of the interaction that marks normal cognitive functioning. Impulses flow in both directions along the fibers of the corpus callosum and other conduits between the two hemispheres to orchestrate their activities. If independent action were more significant than cooperation, it should be easy to carry out two mental tasks simultaneously, one in the left hemisphere and one in the right. In fact, a person with a healthy, intact brain can rarely perform such a feat. The norm is to behave, Milner remarks, like a "single-channel organism."

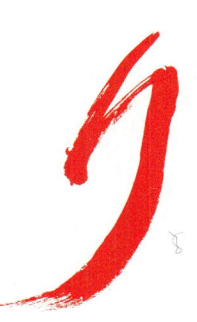

Birds of a feather
The Japanese character above, borrowed from Chinese, signifies bird. But the same word can be spelled using a syllabic alphabet unique to the Japanese language (right). Some researchers believe that the Japanese brain processes the two systems in different regions of the cerebral cortex.

WORDS AND PICTURES

As this sentence is being read, networks of cortical neurons are busily communicating in the brain's left hemisphere. Yet, certain researchers claim that if the text were written in Japanese, readers who had learned that language at a young age would experience synaptic firing in both cerebral hemispheres.

This controversial theory is based on the fact that Japanese writing intermingles two conceptually different writing systems. *Kanji* represents ideas or things in picture form; *kana*, adding one linguistic step, assembles words from individual symbols each representing a vocal syllable.

Adherents of the theory reason that, whereas the left hemisphere processes phonetic symbols such as *kana* syllabics or Roman letters, the right hemisphere takes greater charge of pictures that carry immediate meaning.

Of Two Minds

The subject looks at the midpoint of a screen displaying two images—a sphere on the left side, a cube on the right. When asked what she sees, the woman acknowledges only half the data: "I see one image—a cube." Next, she is asked to use her left hand to feel a few objects hidden behind the screen—including both the cube and the sphere—then to choose the item portrayed on the screen. Curiously, her left hand ignores the cube. Without a word she picks up the sphere.

This epileptic patient has undergone a last-resort operation—severing the corpus callosum, or bridge, between the cerebral hemispheres—to diminish her severe seizures. But as a result, her brain has been divided into two autonomous mental structures. Experiments involving "split-brain" subjects shed light on how the brain thinks.

The subject says the screen contains only the cube; yet only information about the sphere reaches her left hand. Keeping in mind that each of the brain's hemispheres processes information about the opposite visual field, the inevitable conclusion is that the left hemisphere can speak of what it sees, but the right hemisphere is mute. In order to articulate information processed on the right side, the brain must be able to pass it to the left. Yet because the communication link is cut, not only is right hemisphere data lost to speech (a left-hemisphere function), but the individual seems unaware of that data.

Equally intriguing is the left hemisphere's desire to make sense of conflicting data. In another split-brain experiment, the left hemisphere is presented with a picture of a chicken claw while the right hemisphere is shown a scene of winter snow. Asked to choose related images from a number of pictures, the subject correctly points to a chicken with the right hand and a shovel with the left. Chicken and claw form a logical match in the left hemisphere, as do shovel and snow in the right. But since the left hemisphere is unaware of the snow scene, how does the subject justify the shovel verbally? "You need a shovel to clean a chicken shed," he replies.

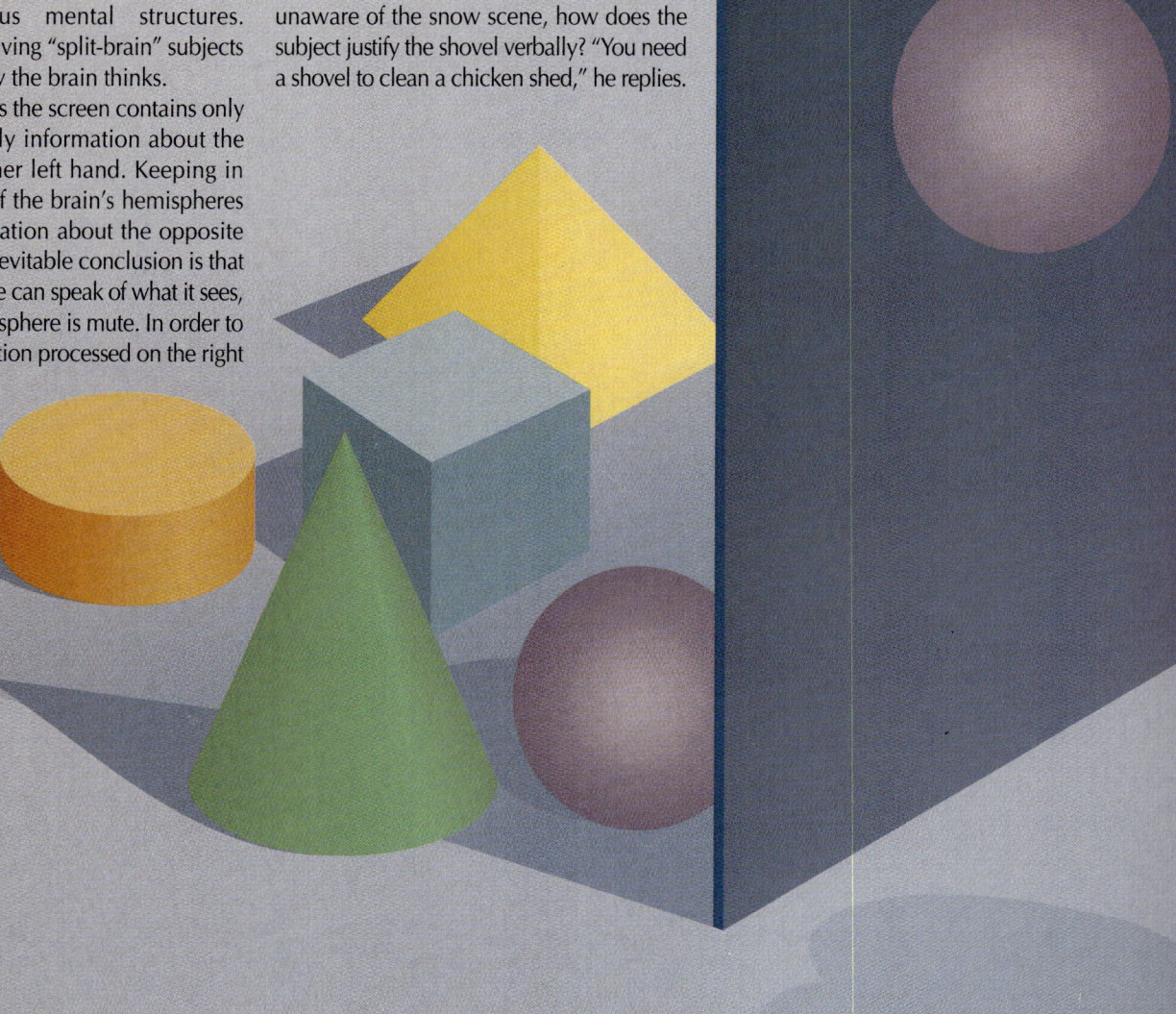

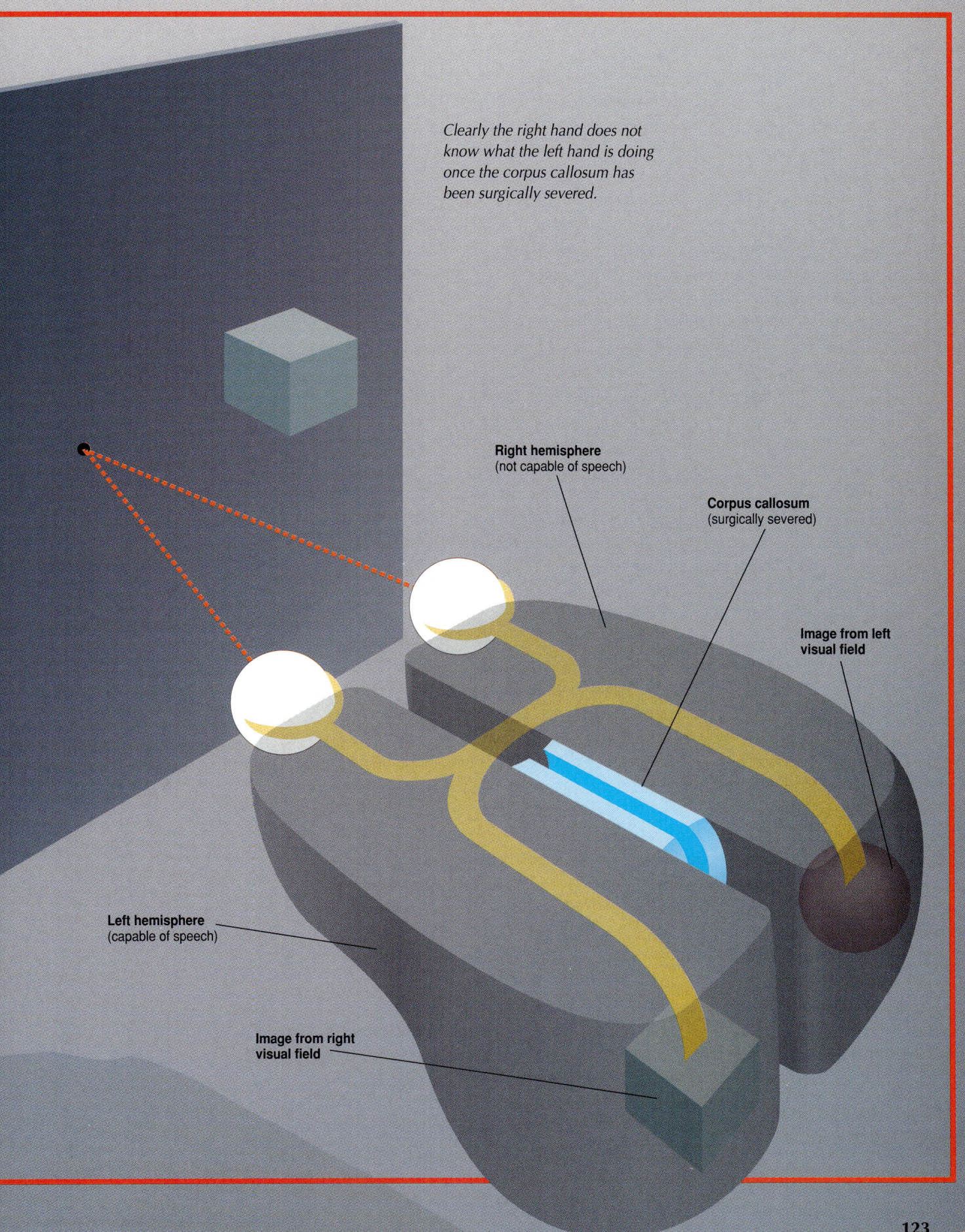

LEAPING LOGIC

The topmost layer of the two hemispheres—the rumply quarter-inch-thick cerebral cortex—coordinates a grab-bag of processes collectively labeled thought. Although not easy to define, thought—conscious and unconscious as well—embraces logic, judgment, comparison, generalization, creativity, learning, memory, concept formation, insight and intuition, planning, a grasp of consequences and problem-solving. Logic, often identified with thinking, is only one mode of thought, and is not always useful. There seems to be a universal tendency to take particular instances and convert them into generalities. Generalizations from personal experience are not rational propositions, but they are often better guides than logic in making a decision.

Human beings, of course, are not the only creatures capable of logical thought. Some animals grasp relationships between objects and events and adapt their behavior accordingly. In an experiment that earned fame for a brainy chimpanzee, a banana was suspended well out of its reach in a small room containing nothing else but a box. The chimpanzee tried jumping for the prize, then in a stroke of ape genius pushed the box under it, climbed up and ate his reward. Pigeons, belying the epithet "birdbrain," can analyze unusual situations and come up with advantageous solutions. Normally groundfeeders, they can be taught to eat food suspended within easy reach, or to use a box exactly as the chimpanzee did to reach a banana hung out of reach. Thinking sometimes comes into play even when there is no obvious benefit. Monkeys have been noted to focus willingly on puzzles whether or not the activity earns them anything tangible, as if problem-solving in itself were the reward.

It is intriguing to speculate how an animal represents its thoughts to itself. In humans, language reports on the brain's decision-making and computations, and the two phenomena are so intricately related that it is sometimes claimed that thought is impossible without language. However, sensory representation is the only way to solve certain kinds of problems. In one test, the subjects were asked to study side-by-side pictures of a pair of three-dimensional geometrical figures and decide whether they were identical. Researchers discovered that the subjects rotated one figure in imagination, exactly as if it were an object in space, so that they could compare it from various points of view to the other figure. From the length of time it took for subjects to solve the problem, scientists were able to determine the rate at which the mental image rotated—about 60 degrees per second. The thinking of deaf people who learn sign language in infancy may rely heavily on visual and spatial forms. Studies hint that these people arrange the stages of a complicated logical problem spatially instead of in the temporal order that hearing people use.

Neuroscientists distinguish between the actual processes of cognition and what is processed. They propose that memory is stocked with mental representations. The stuff of processing, these are representations of external events and objects that the brain constructs from sensory input. Such a mental representation may generate an image quite faithful to the original—the Eiffel Tower, for instance. Others are composite representations that the mind builds over time by abstracting common characteristics from related sensory experiences. The concept "dog" is more schematic than the mental object of Eiffel Tower since it embraces chi-

FACE BY NUMBERS

Computers are veritably blind when it comes to recognizing even as celebrated a visage as this. But in the time required to read this caption, a computer could tally all the numbers painting Mona Lisa's face. The brain, on the other hand, though comparatively weak at mathematics, can instantly recognize the world's most enigmatic face.

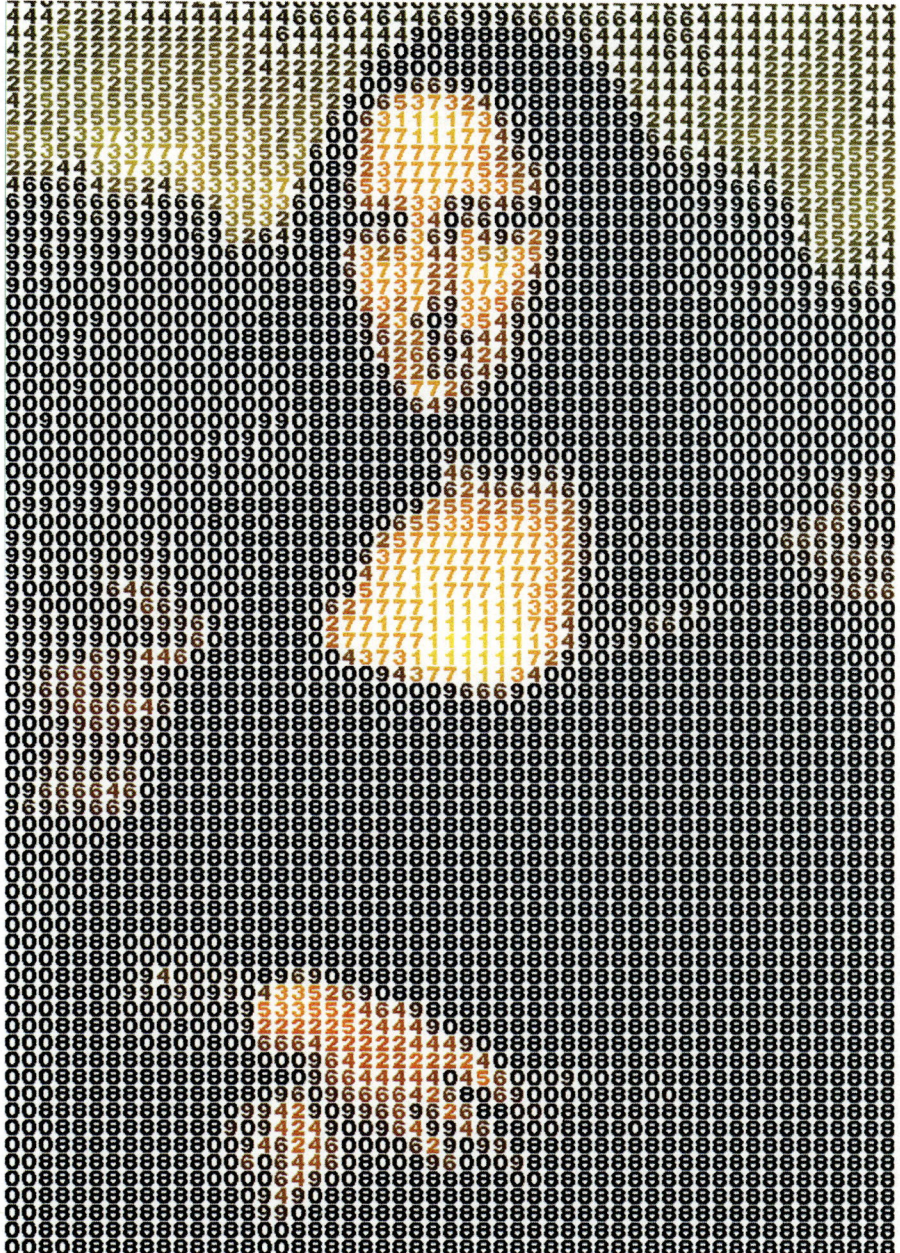

huahuas and mastiffs alike. Interests, needs and point of view help a concept. A geneticist's notion of dog might indicate its differences from wolves, but a layman's sketchier abstraction serves perfectly well. Many mental representations have no sensory referent at all. A four-year-old, asked to name the opposite of "tiger," might reply, "not-tiger." The concept is valid, and at the same time literally unimaginable.

Though the name implies something that occupies a single position in space, French neuroscientist Jean-Pierre Changeux points out that a mental representation is in all likelihood a "delocalized" phenomenon, more an event than a representation. What has been discovered about brain architecture and function suggests that each of these representations is encoded as a particular pattern of chemical and electrical activity in an assembly of cortical cells. Although no method has yet been devised for observing such processes in human neurons, the assembly's synaptic connections probably undergo changes similar to those observed in the marine snail experiments.

Anatomical studies, experiments and observations made in dealing with the effects of injury all indicate that mental representations are processed in the cortex of the frontal lobe. Exploding gunpowder drove an iron bar through the frontal lobes of a New England railroad worker named Phineas Gage who spent the next 12 years under the care of John Harlow; the observant physician made Gage a textbook case. The grievous wound obviously did not harm Gage's frontal lobe centers for language or motor activity. Within an hour of the explosion, he was able to walk to a surgeon's office and describe the accident. Harlow reported, however, that the accident made Gage "capricious and vacillating, devising many plans of future operation, which no sooner are arranged than they are abandoned in favor of others he finds more practical." Along with losing his ability to organize his life, Gage lost the ability to judge and regulate his behavior. He became "fitful and irreverent," profane and profoundly indifferent to other people's feelings.

No aspect of thought is safe from frontal-lobe injury or disease. Temporal judgment may suffer, making it impossible to recall either the frequency of events or the order in which they occurred. No new "time-tagged" memories can be stored, and planning a sequence of activities—even one as simple as stringing beads in a particular color sequence—becomes impossible. Concentration, abstract reasoning, problem-solving and creativity are equally vulnerable, and emotional factors such as the curiosity that drives the engines of intellectual activity dissipate.

The massive bundles of nerve fibers connecting the frontal cortex to the parietal, occipital and temporal cortices deliver highly refined information based on touch, smell and taste, vision and hearing, and sensations from within the body itself. Moreover, the connections are reciprocal: Far from being passive, the frontal lobe influences the analytical activity of the other three lobes. Besides their links to the frontal lobe, the parietal, occipital and temporal lobes communicate directly with one another through a spider's web of fibers. Axons stretching from one lobe to another are connected to the target's association area. Here, sensory information that has already been processed at lower levels is refined again into an abstract perceptual package, or mental representation.

The frontal cortex receives a continual stream of these representations. It integrates this fresh information with what is called "re-entrant" information—relevant memories summoned from the limbic system—and with emotional input, which also arrives via the limbic system. As a result of the integration, the frontal cortex may plot an overt motor action—speech or a calculated movement—or trigger a purely mental event such as an unexpressed thought or a complex image.

PET scans paint with a broad brush the ebb and flow of blood in the perceiving, thinking human brain, but implanted probes are beginning to locate more exactly the neurons that mediate thought. Electrical activity has been recorded in the macaque monkey's frontal lobe during a "delayed-response" task. As the monkey watches, a piece of food is placed under one of two identical bowls that are out of reach. After a few minutes' delay the monkey is allowed to approach the bowls and choose the one it thinks covers the food. A snack rewards the right choice. Each stage of the test showed its own particular pattern of neuronal activity. In the monkeys who remembered where the food had been hidden, certain neurons

NETWORKS OF BRILLIANCE

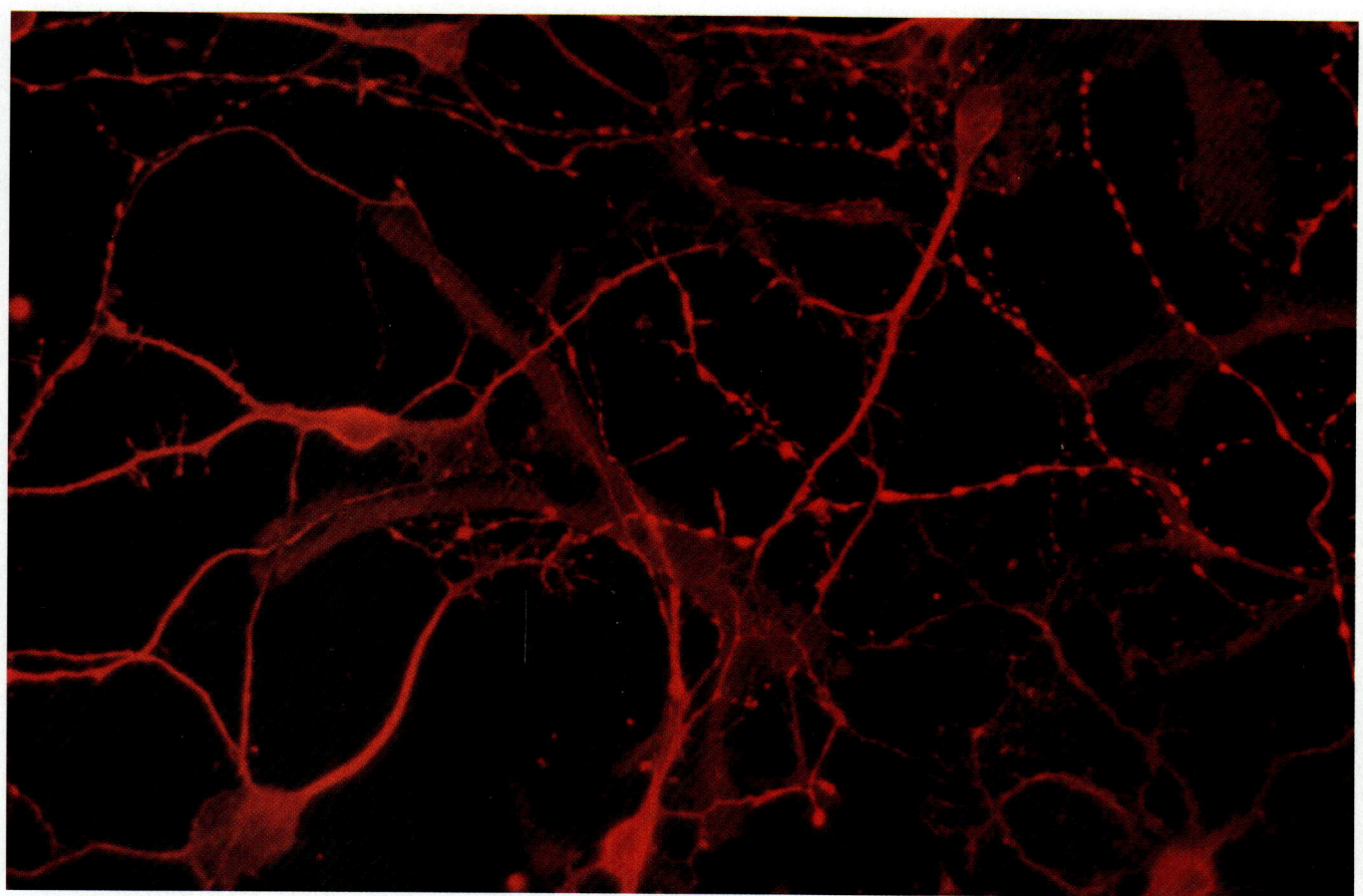

A neural network appears to glow with electricity, thanks to a special fluorescent dye. Normally a nondescript mélange of white and gray, nerve cells are prepared with a variety of treatments to render them more visible.

stepped up their rate of firing after the monkeys had watched the food being hidden. Those neurons stayed active throughout the delay period, until the monkey was freed to choose a bowl. But the activity of the same neurons in a forgetful monkey showed no change during the delay period. The probes had apparently detected neurons in the very act of storing what the monkey had seen and forming a plan to get the food.

Though all the test subjects set about their task under identical circumstances and were given identical information, their performances were not identical. Monitoring showed that the same areas of the frontal cortex were activated in all of the monkeys, so they presumably attacked the task with the same perceptual and cognitive processes. But some monkeys were much quicker to discover a relationship between a choice that earned them a reward and what they had seen the experimenter do with the bowls and food.

The capacity to discover such associations and to learn from experience demonstrates intelligence, according to most definitions. Monkeys—and humans—also reveal their intelligence when they make advantageous changes in behavior in response to changes in their surroundings.

GRADE A BRAIN

It is easy to detect the results of intelligence, but very difficult to pin down what the word means. Philosophers have argued about the nature of intelligence for centuries, but the debate took on a more scientific cast during the 19th Century

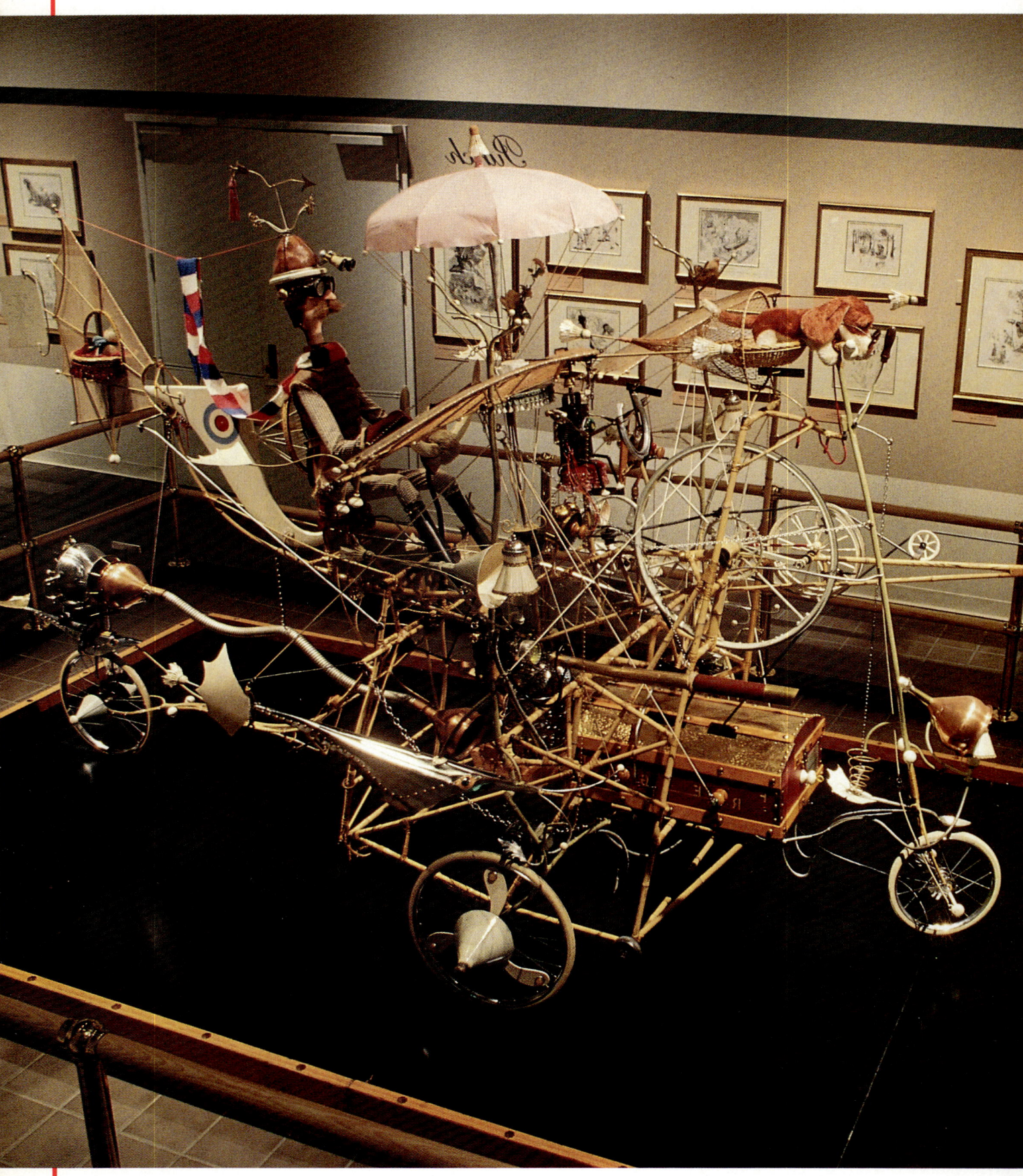

NETWORK OF BRILLIANCE

Free Thinking

The ability to think creatively is most often regarded as a talent possessed by the "gifted." Yet, like typing or driving a car, creative thinking depends on method, the result of learning and practice. Every brain possesses a reservoir of creative ability, ready to be applied to projects and problems from the marvelous to the mundane.

Most Westerners are unconsciously schooled in a form of linear analysis descended from Greek logic: If A=B and B=C, then A=C. But rational thinking is not always equal to the task at hand.

Original, creative thinking leaps off the rails of straight-line reasoning, linking ideas in surprising patterns. The association areas of the cerebral cortex, vast interconnections of neural networks, link related data automatically. A less rigid approach to reasoning reveals wild and wonderful relationships between ideas and things that are the essence of creative discovery.

Innovative artists and scientists, as well as creative people enthused with the challenges of everyday living, suggest the following ideas and techniques to broaden conventional horizons:

Define a problem as broadly and confidently as possible. A solution already exists and is only awaiting discovery. Example: The mosquitoes at the cottage must be dealt with.

Next, freely list as many solutions as possible, without judging their plausibility—at this stage there is no risk of failure.

1. Install a family of bug-eating bats in the attic of the cottage.
2. Drain the lake to destroy the mosquitoes' nesting ground.
3. Lure the insects away by dropping a bloody steak in the neighbors' yard.

In seeking possible solutions, break loose from tired patterns of thinking by seeing the situation from an unusual angle. Imagine a dialogue with a turncoat mosquito spy, willing to divulge his comrades' weaknesses.

Avoid settling on a solution at too early a stage. Premature rejection or acceptance of ideas prevents the brain from rolling up its sleeves and tackling the question in earnest. All creative thinkers describe a so-called "incubation" period in which attention is diverted elsewhere. The brain—its neurons stocked with a host of possibilities—is left unhindered to combine networks in ways the conscious vision might miss. The period of distraction can last from minutes to years, depending on circumstances and the scope of the problem. Then...

Eureka! A solution presents itself. Use a steak, but instead of giving it to the mosquitoes in a neighbor's yard, barbecue it, driving away all tiny winged pests with charcoal smoke.

Of course, the well-trained creative thinker becomes attuned to murmurs of doubt—the result, once again, of associated neural activity—and may now rely on dry logic to continue the plan: Since the blood-thirsty mosquitoes will return for the kill just as the dinner bell sounds, continue the smoke assault, burning dead leaves, grass and twigs throughout the meal.

Oh yes; equip everyone with gas masks!

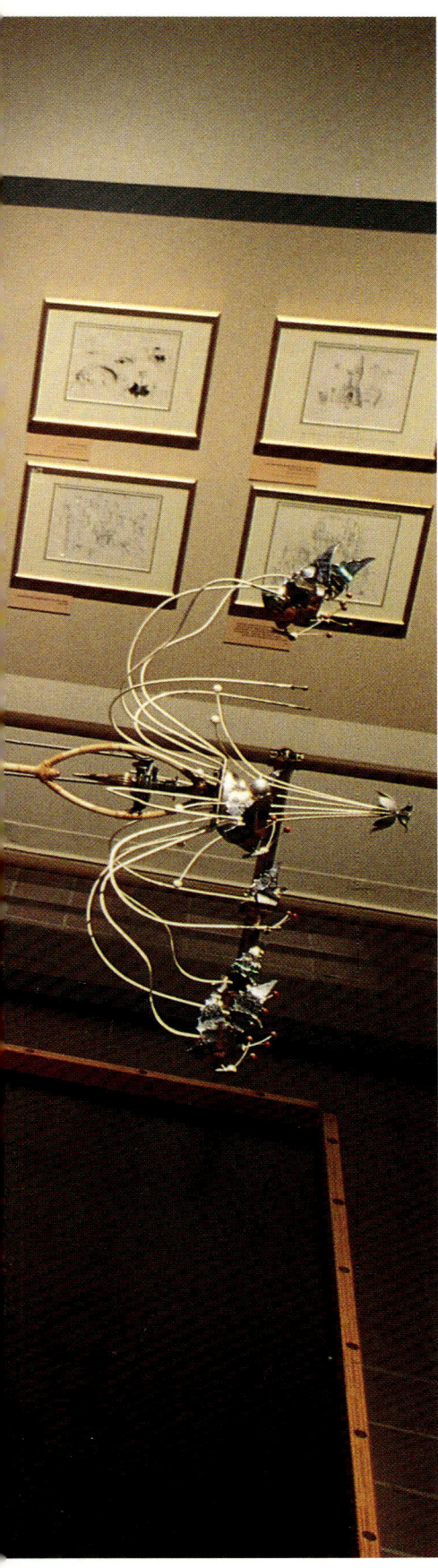

Inventor-artist Rowland Emett frees his mind from the constraints of conventional thinking to create such friendly parodies of the mechanistic age as this one, entitled Fred, Piloting the Featherstone Kite.

Giant Steps

At the turn of the 19th Century a flamboyant Viennese anatomist named Franz Joseph Gall turned heads with his technique for localizing brain function. Gall called his "science" phrenology, and for nearly a century it fascinated both Europe and the New World by professing to predict abilities and traits by noting specific cranial bumps and hollows. Gall had the right idea; brain function can be localized. Marvelous scanning techniques now clearly show areas of neural activity for both function and thought. But Gall never could have foreseen how far the science of the brain would progress in just one century.

The last 15 years alone have seen more discoveries about the brain than in all of history. Ten years ago very few neurotransmitters had been identified. Today more than 40 are known. Understanding the chemical role each plays in the body is essential if we are to correct imbalances and relieve symptoms of diseases such as Huntington's chorea, Parkinson's and Alzheimer's, mental retardation and schizophrenia. The next 10 years will bring detailed understanding of even more neurotransmitters and of how they interrelate to ensure normal and healthy functioning of the brain.

The next 10 years also will see an explosion in the field of pharmacology. Each degree of increased understanding of how the brain and its chemicals work opens up the possibility for more specifically targeted drugs—drugs that will bind exactly where they are meant to and that, because of their specificity, will create far fewer unwanted side effects.

Brain implants and neuron regeneration are at the leading edge of current research and along with the exploding field of genetic engineering will bring the human race face to face with possibilities that until now existed only in the realm of science fiction. Society very soon will be faced with unprecedented ethical and moral questions. What will human beings do with their new-found ability to create genetically 'perfect' people, or with their advance knowledge that a certain child, still in its mother's womb, will be born with a mental or physical defect?

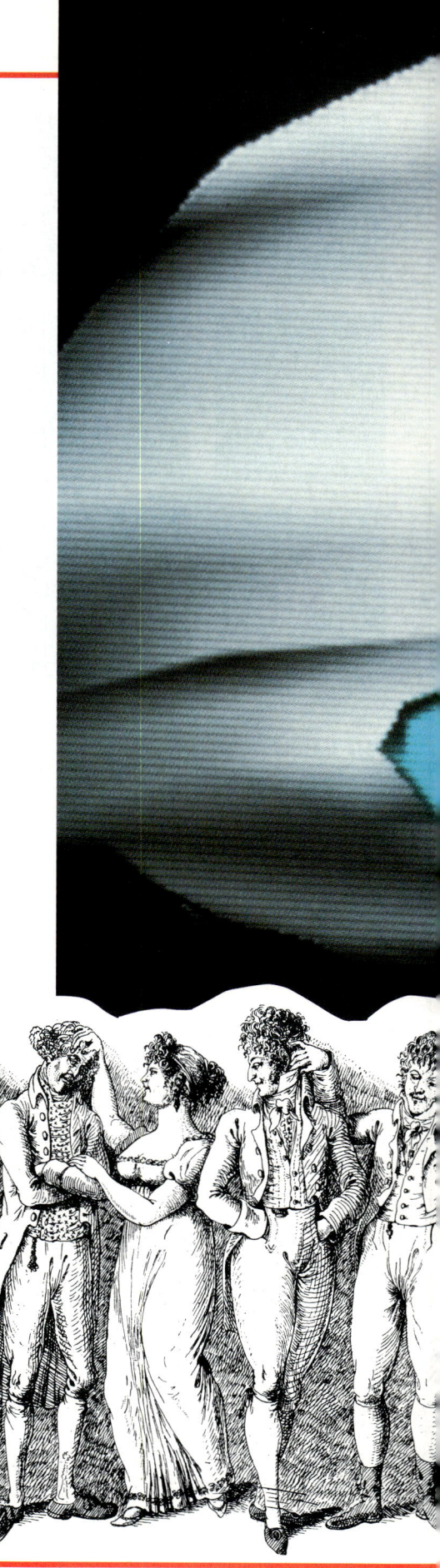

A tongue-in-cheek caricature of the 19th Century shows European society's full-blown devotion to phrenology—the supposed science of feeling skulls for assessment of character. The head was divided into at least 100 areas such as "cautiousness," "sublimity" and "conjugal love."

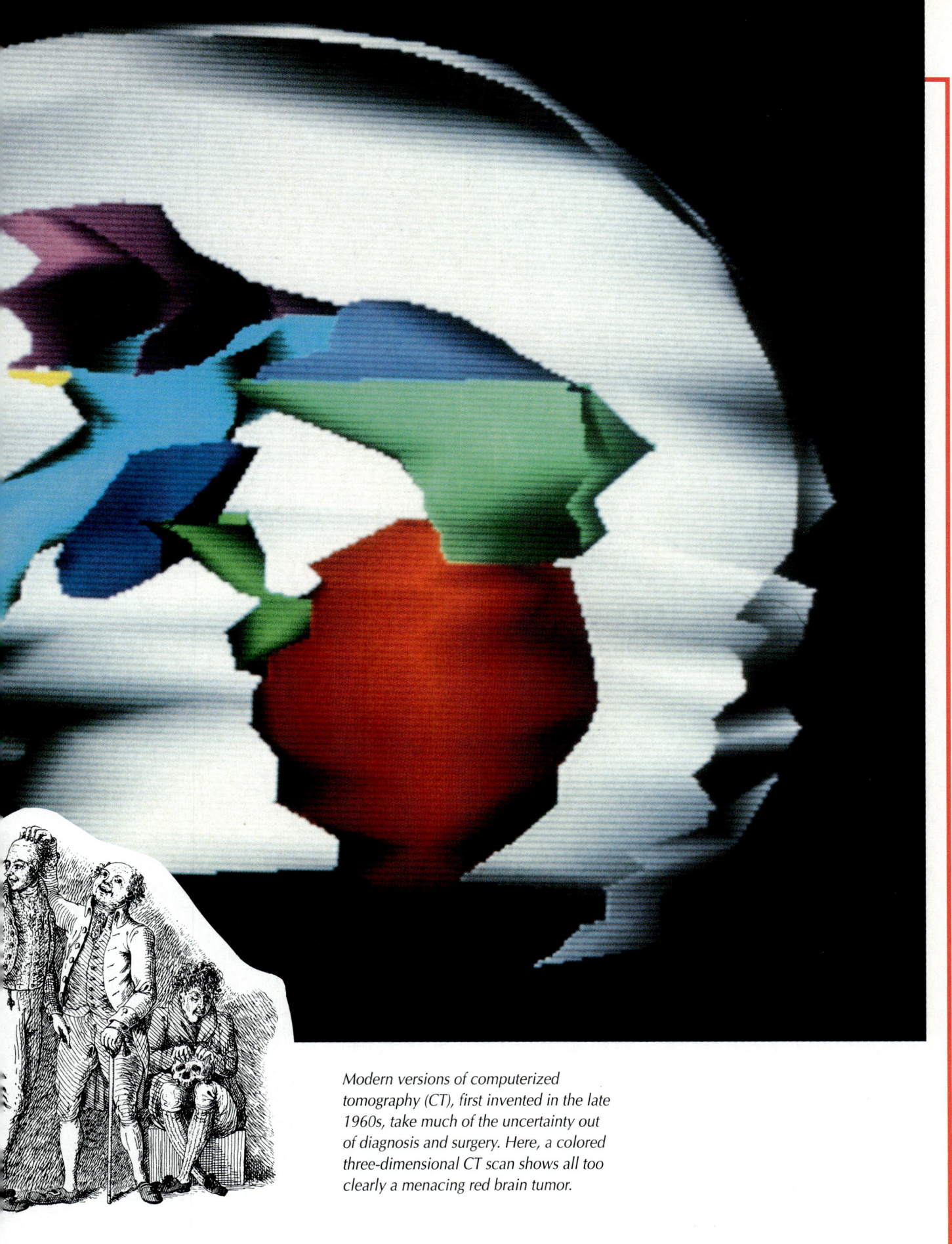

Modern versions of computerized tomography (CT), first invented in the late 1960s, take much of the uncertainty out of diagnosis and surgery. Here, a colored three-dimensional CT scan shows all too clearly a menacing red brain tumor.

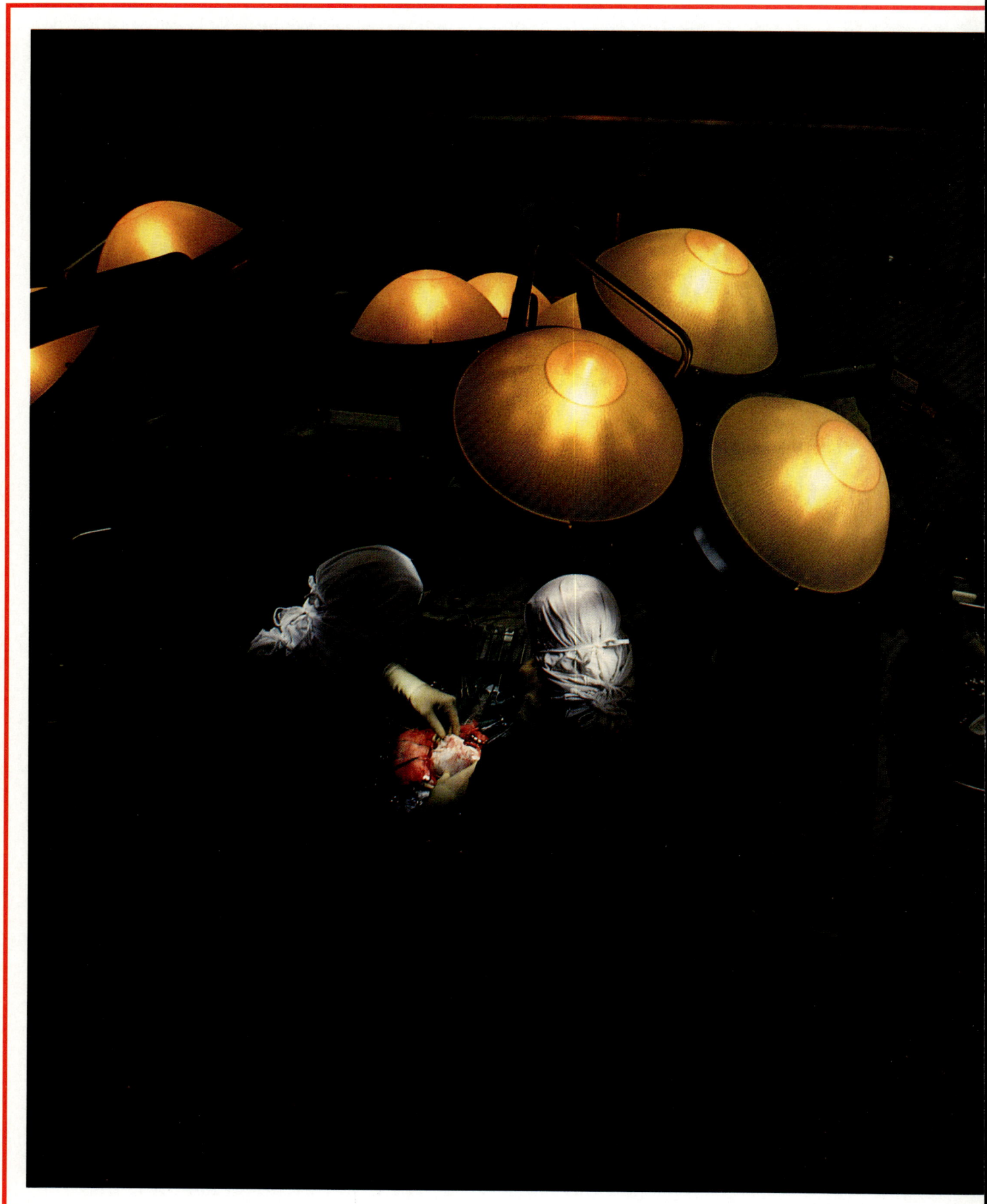

Brain cells do not regenerate. Once destroyed by trauma, disease or disorder, they are lost forever. Or so went neurology's conventional wisdom. But in a remarkable reversal, researchers are discovering ways to restore lost function to brain cells. Injuries and diseases previously considered untreatable may soon respond to new neural implant and regeneration techniques as the processes move from labs to hospitals.

Animal research has already shown that implanted cells not only grow and form connections with existing brain cells, but also that they can replace damaged or destroyed nerve cells in some of the most cruel mental disorders. Humans afflicted with hereditary neurological diseases also have received implants—from other parts of their own brains and from fetal tissue donations.

Sweden and Mexico have gained some impressive sucessses in relatively young Parkinson victims by implanting in the brain tissue from the patient's own adrenal medullae, which sit atop the kidneys. These cells produce dopamine, lacking in Parkinson victims because the dopamine-producing cells in their brains mysteriously die off.

Though neuroscientists seem to have uncorked a genie, they are not really sure how the magic works. Does the implant stimulate remaining brain cells to resume dopamine production? Does the graft itself produce the neurotransmitter? Or does the shock of implant surgery provoke the beneficial response?

In test animals with Huntington's chorea, fetal neural tissue has been used to replace the unhealthy caudate nucleus, which is responsible for smooth, coordinated movements; new neural connections were made. Fetal neurons containing brain chemicals that are associated with memory have dramatically improved the way aged rats perform on memory tests. Alzheimer patients also might benefit from implants.

As well as the concern about "harvesting" fetal tissue, there is the question of whether brain cell implants may transform a recipient. Is the brain being changed by the foreign cells? Animal research indicates that for small implants, the receiving brain takes over new tissue. But larger tissue implants may turn out to have a different effect.

In the exciting field of trophic factors—naturally occurring substances that encourage cells to grow and regenerate—the most studied is nerve growth factor. A mixture of hormones and nutrients, NGF is used to bathe damaged cells. In the lab it stimulates regrowth and regeneration. The next hurdle is to learn whether the regrown nerve will make the right connections. Then there is the problem of how to insert the NGF into the brains of living patients. But considering the pace of progress in the last decade alone, solutions cannot be far off.

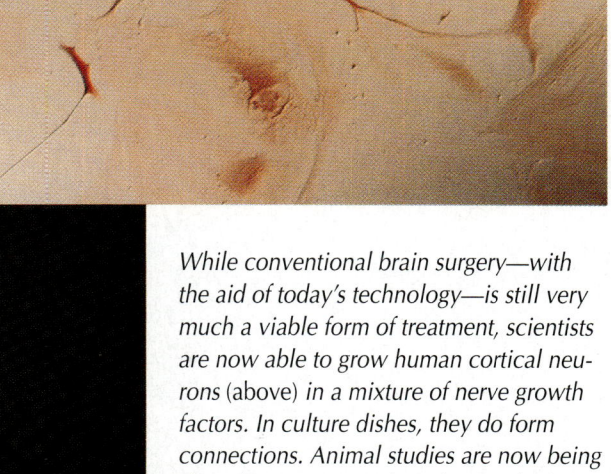

While conventional brain surgery—with the aid of today's technology—is still very much a viable form of treatment, scientists are now able to grow human cortical neurons (above) *in a mixture of nerve growth factors. In culture dishes, they do form connections. Animal studies are now being done, but it is too early to know whether the cells will be able to repopulate a damaged human brain.*

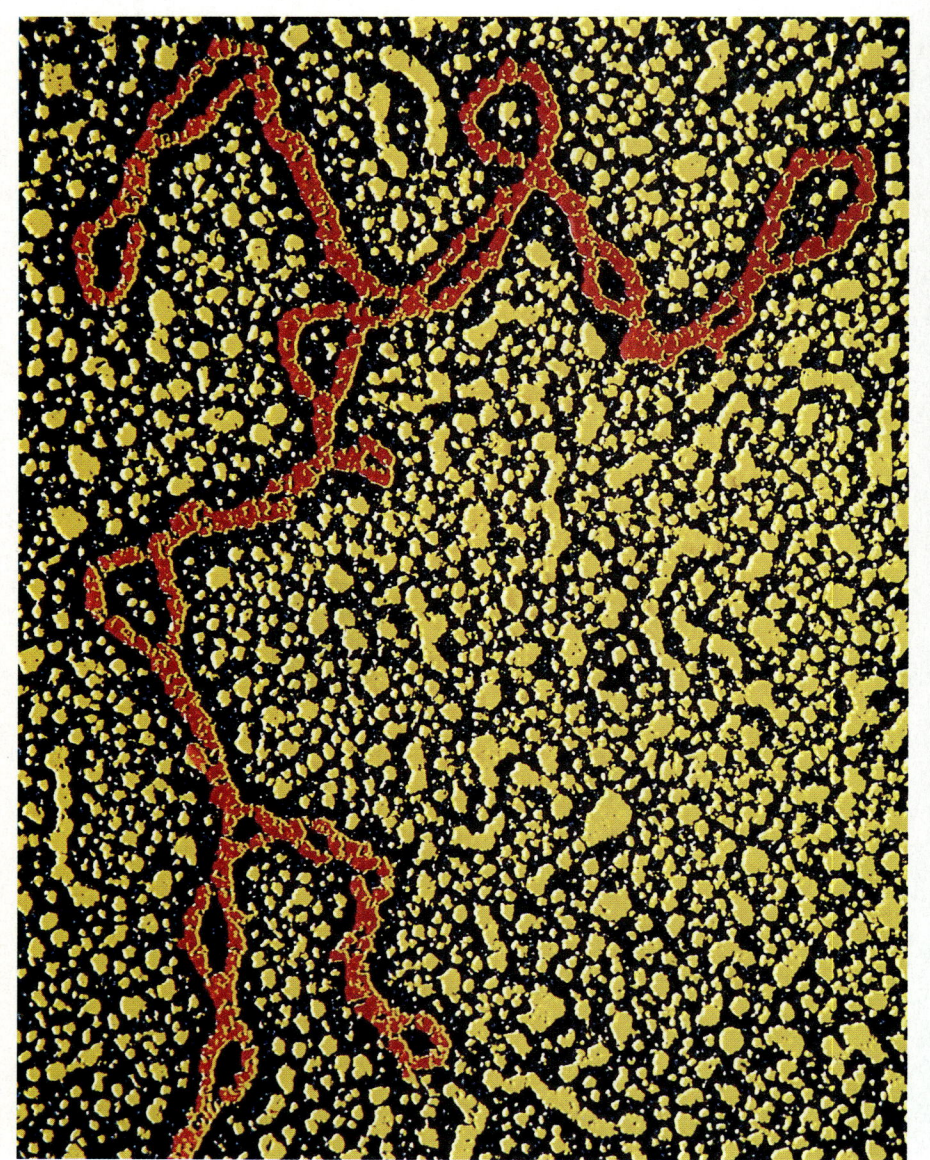

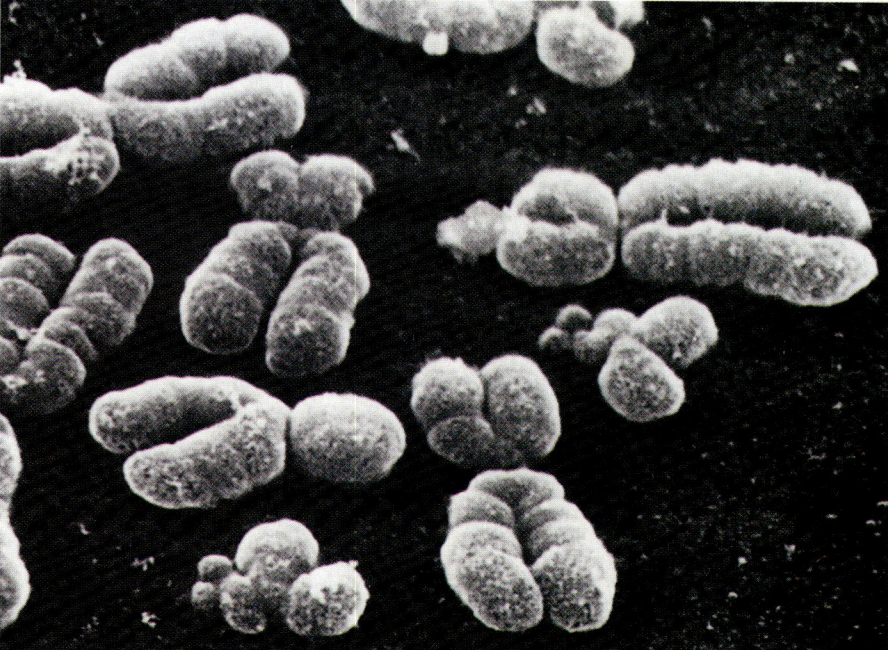

A false-color micrograph (above) shows DNA from a mitochondrion—a structure found in the jelly-like cytoplasm that surrounds the nucleus of all plant and animal cells. At right are human chromosomes. The smallest human chromosome contains about 5,000 genes, all of which are simply DNA segments. A researcher (opposite page) studies bands of DNA in a solution that causes them to fluoresce.

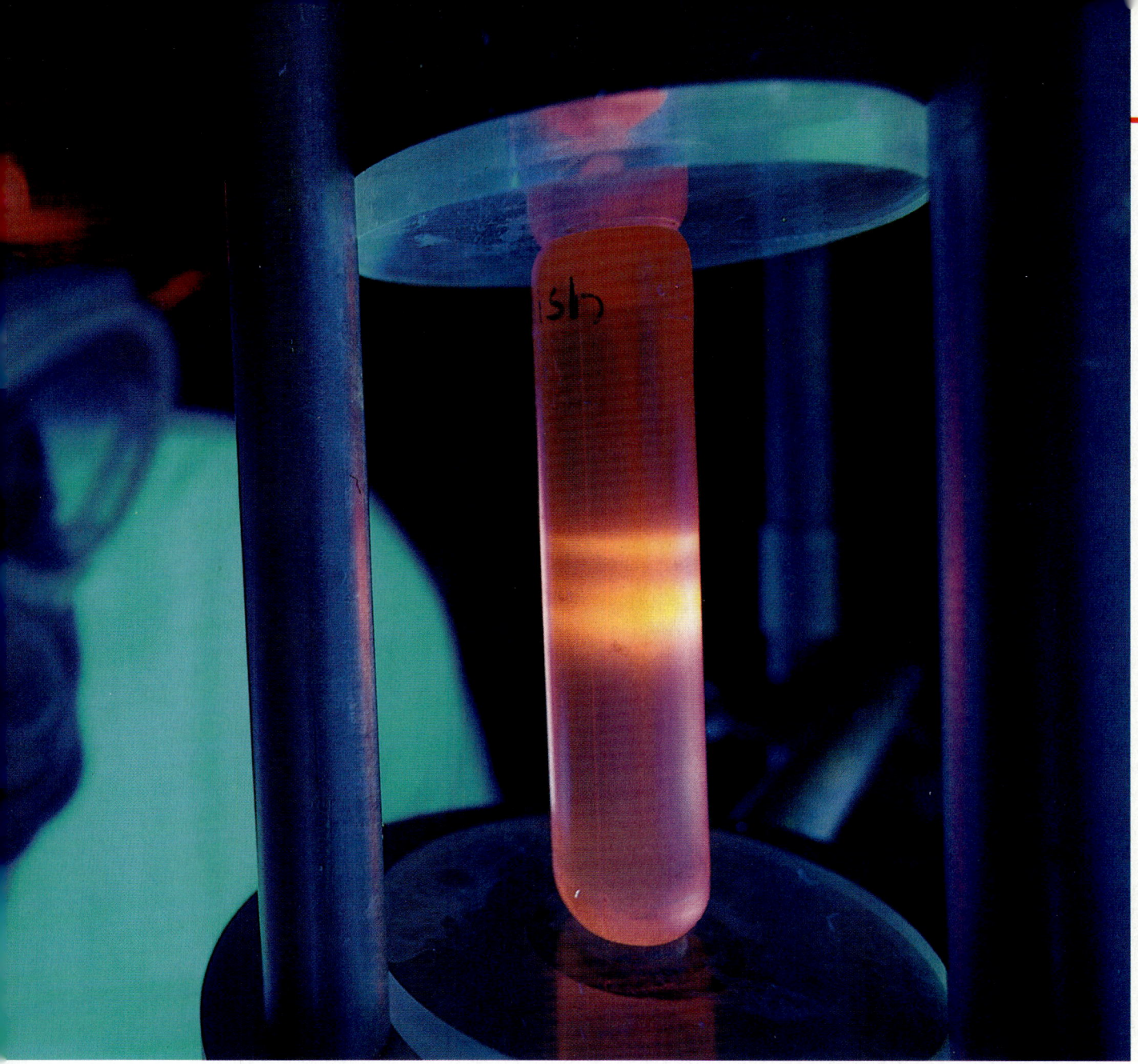

Before 1953, almost no one had heard the term DNA. But that year two young research scientists named James Watson and Francis Crick put those three letters on the map when they plotted the structure of the material from which all genes are made. In chemical terms the letters stand for deoxyribonucleic acid, but in everyday parlance DNA is the building block of all life.

The human genome—23 pairs of chromosomes (23 from each parent)— contains every bit of data needed to make a human being. Genes are part of chromosomes, which themselves are largely composed of long strands of DNA. Only four chemical bases—adenine, cytosine, guanine and thymine (A,C,G and T)—run along the length of each DNA molecule, but the order in which they are combined is a code that tells the cells to produce the proteins necessary to make eyes blue or blood cells round. It almost defies the powers of human understanding to realize that the whole story of life is written with only a four-letter alphabet.

From beginning to end, the book of life is thought to be three billion letters long. And somewhere in that book—on one line of one page of one chapter—lies the answer to any genetic disease. Scientists are deciphering the human genome, gene by gene, in an effort to identify the defective genetic sequences associated with inherited disorders.

When these diseases have common symptoms, the search for defects is less painstaking. Scientists, noting that older Down's syndrome patients develop Alzheimer-like symptoms, searched chromosome 21 (associated with Down's) for a clue to the cause of Alzheimer's. Once genes are implicated, it then may be possible to use DNA probes. Probes bind with complementary strands of DNA and help detect both active and inactive genes. A patient could be told that he is the carrier of a gene for a disease that he could pass on to offspring, or that he will himself develop the disease. Genetic abnormalities may also underlie illnesses such as schizophrenia and manic depression.

Index

Numerals in *italics* indicate an illustration of the subject mentioned.

A

Acetylcholine, 40, 60, 69, 102, 117
Addictions, 98-105, *98, 99, 101, 103*
  Endorphins, 99, 104
Adrenal glands, 24, 92, 137
Adrenaline, 24, 92, 98
Adrenocorticotrophin (ACTH), 93
Aggressive behavior, 76-78, 81
Alcoholism, 102-*103*
Alexia, 119
Alkon, Dr. Daniel L., 114
Alzheimer's disease, *116-117*, 134, 137, 139
Amphetamines, 98, *99, 103*
Amygdala, 81, 95, 108, 112
  Removal, 81, 108, 112
Amyloid, *116-117*
Androgens, 40, *41*, 42, 43
Antidepressants, 83, 86
Anxiety. *See* Stress
Aphasia, 119
Aphrodisiacs, 43, 84
  Aplysia, 106, 113-115, *114-115*
Arcuate fasciculus, 119
Aristotle, 14, 79
Aserinsky, Eugene, 56, 67
Association cortex, 53
Astrocytes, 18, *19*
Auditory cortex, 16, 28
Auditory system. *See* Hearing
Autism, *131*, 132
Autonomic nervous system, 22-23, 26
  Sexual behavior, 42, 43
  See also Parasympathetic nervous system; Sympathetic nervous system
Axons, 18-21, *18, 20*

B

Balance, 33, 37
Basal ganglia, 37, 38
  Parkinson's disease, *38-39*
Besedovsky, Dr. Hugo, 94
Beta blockers, 95
Binet, Alfred, 130
Biochemistry:
  Emotions, 82-83, 86
Biofeedback, 59
Brain, 14, *16-17, 117*
  Development, *8-13*
  Weight, Size, *10*
  See also names of specific parts of the brain
Brain cells. *See* Neurons
Brainstem, *17*, 80
  Dreaming, 67
  Sleep, 57, 60

Brainwaves, *54-55*, 57
  Psychological depression, 66
Broca, Pierre Paul, 118-119
  Quoted, 119
Broca's area, 119, *120*

C

Cade, Dr. John, 82-83
Cannon, Walter, 79
Central nervous system (CNS), 22, 23
  Stimulants, 103
Cerebellum, *13, 16-17, 37*, 40
Changeux, Jean-Pierre, 125
Chernobyl nuclear accident, 62
Children:
  Brain development, *8-13*
  Interneurons, 22
  Language acquisition, 118, 121
  REM sleep, 66, 72
  Sexual dimorphism, 40-43
Chimpanzees, 115
Chlorpromazine, 91
Chomsky, Noam, 118
Chromosome 21, 117, *138*, 139
Cingulate gyrus, *78*, 79-80
Circadian rhythms, 60-63
  Insomnia, 69
  Jet lag, *64-65*
  Napping, *74-75*
  Sleep laboratories, *74-75*
Classical conditioning, 114
Cocaine, 100-103, *101, 103*
Cochlea, 32-33
Color blindness, 28
Comas, 55
Communication, 106
Computerized tomography (CT), 44, *135*
Congenital disorders, 132, 139
Consciousness, 52-56, *52-53*
  Emotions, 78
  See also Thought
Corpus callosum, *17*, 53, 55-56, 119
  Split-brain operations, 55-56, *122-123*
Cortex, 9, 11, *12, 16-17*, 98, 106, *112-113, 120*, 121
  Dreaming, 67
  Gustatory, *16*
  See also Laterality
Cortisol, 93-94
Creativity, *128-129*, 130-131
Crick, Francis, 139
  Quoted, 133

D

Declarative knowledge, 109, 112, 114
Defense mechanisms, 26-27
de Frutos, Jesus, 69
Dement, William, 57
Dendrites, *12*, 18, *20*, 21
  Sensitization, 114
Deoxyribonucleic acid (DNA), *138-139*
Depression, 79, 82-83, *86*, 87
  Cortisol, 93-94
  Manic depression, 82-83, *86-87*

REM sleep, 66, 72
Seasonal affective disorder (SAD), 86
Depth perception, 28, 30
Descartes, René, 50
  Quoted, 52
Diagnostic tools:
  Computerized tomography (CT), *135*
  Magnetic resonance imagery (MRI), 44-46, *44-45*
  Magnetoencephalography (MEG), *48-49*
  Positron emission tomography (PET), 46-48, *46-47*, 120
Diamond, Marian, 132
Dickinson, Emily:
  Quoted, 79, 91
Diffuse enteric nervous system, 26
Digestive system, 26
Diseases:
  Detection, *44-49*, 139
Dopamine, 91, *98, 99*, 137
  Drug abuse and, 100-102, *101*
  Love, 84
  Malfunctions, 38, 69, 91, 137
Down's syndrome, 117, 139
Dreaming, 57, 67-73, *70-71, 72*
  Brainwaves, *54-55*
  Meaning, 73
  Non-REM sleep, 57, 60, 66
  See also REM sleep
Drugs, 55, 134
  Abuse, 55, 100-*103*
  See also Medications
Dualism, 50
Dystonia, 40

E

Eardrums, 32
Ears. *See* Hearing
Elderly people: *12-13*
  Sleep, 66
Electroencephalogram (EEG), *54-55*
Elkes, Dr. Joel:
  Quoted, 93
Emotions, 79
  Biochemistry, 82-83, 86
  Happiness, *96-97*
  Love, *84-85*
  See also Limbic system
Endorphins, 42, 98-100, *101*, 104
  Laughter, 97
  Love, 84
  Stress, 98-100
Enkephalins, 98-100, 104
Environment:
  Heredity and, 103, 130, 132
Epilepsy, 48, 55-56, 81
Epinephrine, 92
Estrogen, *40-41*, 42
Euphoria, 81, 84, 104
  Drug induced, 98, 100, 102
  Sexual activity, 42
Exercise, 104
Eyes. *See* Vision

140

INDEX

F-G
Facial expressions, *76-77*, *88-89*
Fetus, *8-9*
Feelings. *See* Emotions
Fight-or-flight response, *24-25*, 92-93
Follicle-stimulating hormone (FSH), 42
Freud, Sigmund, 56
  The Interpretation of Dreams, 73
  Quoted, 78
Frontal lobe, *16*, *36*, 37
  Injury, 126
  See also Motor cortex
GABA, 98, 102
Gage, Phineas, 126
Gall, Franz Joseph, 134
Galton, Sir Francis, 130
Ganglia, 22
Gazzaniga, Michael, 55-56
Gender differences. *See* Sexual dimorphism
Genetic engineering, 134
Genes, 11, 139
Glial cells, 10, 18, *19*
Goodall, Jane:
  Quoted, 115

H
Habituation, 113-114
Happiness, *96-97*
Healing: 97
  Sleep, 63, 66
Hearing, 32-33
  Language perception, 33, 119
  Laterality, 119-120
Heredity: 137, 139
  Environment and, 103, 130, 132
Hippocampus, 80, 93, 94, 108, *109*
Hippocrates, 79
  Quoted, 14
Hobson, J. Allan, 73
Hormones, 26
  Cortisol, 93-94
  Sexual behavior, *40-43*
  Sleep, 63, 66
  See also Neurotransmitters
Hughes, Dr. John, 98-99
Huntington's chorea, 38, 134, 137
Hypothalamus, *17*, *23*, 26, 53, 80, 81, 95, 53
  Aggressive behavior, 76-77
  Olfactory processing, 32
  Sexual behavior, 40, 42
  Sleep, 57, 60
  Stress, 24, 92-93, 94

I
Iconic memory, 112
Idiots savants, *131*-132
Immune system, 26-27, 96
  Stress, 94
Implants, 134, *137*
Insomnia, 60, 66, *68*-69
Instinctual behavior:
  REM sleep, 72-73
Intelligence, 127, 130-133
  Creativity, *128-129*, 130-*131*
  Tests, 130, *133*
Interneurons, 22
Ions, 21
IQ, 130, *131*-132
Isoniazid, 83

J-K
James, William:
  Quoted, 79
Japanese writing, *121*
Jet lag, *64-65*
Jouvet, Michel, 72-73
Judgment, 126
Kandel, Dr. Eric, 113-114
Kleitman, Nathaniel, 56-57, 67
Korsakov's syndrome, 112-113
Kosterlitz, Dr. Hans, 98-99

L
Language, 33, 115
  Children, 118
  Laterality, 118-121, *118-119*, *121*
  Sign language, 118, 121, 124
Laterality, *118-119*
  Autism, *131*, 132
  Facial expressions, *88-89*
  Idiots savants, *131*-132
  Language, 118-121, *118-119*, *121*
  Sensory systems, 53
  Vision, *27*, 29-30, *88-89*, 119
  Split-brain operations, 55-56, *122-123*
Laughter, *96-97*
L-dopa, 38
Learning:
  Classical conditioning, 114
  Habituation, 113-114
  Sensitization, 114
  See also Memory; Motor skills
Left hemisphere, 56, 131
  See also Laterality
Li, C., 98
Light:
  Circadian rhythms, 61, *65*, 69, 86
  Seasonal affective disorder (SAD), 86
  Vision, 28-29
Limbic system, *78*, 80, 83, 126
  Smell, 31, 32
  See also Amygdala; Hippocampus
Lithium carbonate, 82-83
Locus coeruleus, 60, 72, 83, 95
Logic, 12, 124
Love, *84-85*
Luteinizing hormone (LH), 42

M
MacLean, Paul, 80
Magnetic resonance imagery (MRI), 10, *13*, 44-46, *44-45*
Magnetoencephalography (MEG), *48-49*
Mahadevan, Rajan, *111*
Manic depression, 82-83, 86, *87*, 139
McCarley, Robert, 73

Medications:
  Contraceptives, 42
  Depression, 83, 86
  Mania, 82-83
  Parkinson's disease, 38
  Schizophrenia, 91
  Sleep, 66, 69
  Stress, 91-*92*, 98
  See also Drugs
Medulla oblongata, *17*
Melatonin, 61, 86
Memory, 108, *110-111*
  Alzheimer's disease, *116-117*
  Iconic, 112
  Long-term, 112-113
  Mental representations, 124-126
  REM sleep, 73
  Short term, 12, 108-113
  Smell, 31
  Stress, *92*-93
  Taste, 31
Mental illness. *See* Psychological disorders; Names of specific diseases
Milner, Brenda, 108
  Quoted, 121
Monism, 50
Monoamine oxidase (MAO), 83
Moods. *See* Emotions
Morphine, 98, *101*
Motor cortex, *16-17*, 33, 35-37, 40
Motor neurons, *34-35*
Motor skills, 35-37, *36*, 40, 109
Movement, 35-40, *36*
Multiple sclerosis, *18*
Muscles:
  Motor neurons, *34-35*, 40
  REM sleep, 47
Myelin sheaths, 10, *18*, *19*, 21

N
Narcolepsy, 66, 69
Nerve growth factor (NGF), 117, *137*
Neural networks, *127*
Neuroendocrine system, 22, 23, 24
  See also Hypothalamus; Pituitary gland
Neurons, *8-9*, *10-11*, *12-13*, 14-22, *14-15*, *18-21*, 50, *106-107*
  Alzheimer's disease, *116-117*
  Cones, 28-29
  Drug binding, *101*
  Implants, *137*
  Motor, *34-35*
  Motor cortex, *36*
  Regeneration, *134*, *137*
  Rods, 28-29
  Thought, 126-*127*
Neurotransmitters, 21-22, 134
  Aplysia, 115
  Emotions, 82
  Exercise, 104
  Fight-or-flight response, *24-25*
  Learning, 113
  Sleep, 60

Stress, 93-94
See also Hormones
Niacin, 82
Nicklaus, Jack, 95
Nicotine, 103
Night blindness, 28-29
Nightmares, 73
Node of Ranvier, *20*
Noradrenaline, 24, 60, 72, 83
    Love, *84-85*
    Stress, 92
Nuclear medicine:
    Positron emission tomography (PET), 46-48, *46-47*, 120
Nucleus accumbens, *98*, 102

O-P

Occipital lobe, *16*
Occipital cortex. *See* Visual cortex
Olds, Dr. James, 80-81
Olfactory senses. *See* Smell
Oligodendrocytes, *19*
Opiates, 98, *101*, 103
    See also Endorphins
Optical illusions, *26*
Optic nerve, 29-30
Oxytocin, 42
Pain, 35, 93
    Endorphins, 98, 99-100
Panic attacks, *92*, 94-95
Papez, James W., 80
Parasympathetic nervous system, 26
Parkinson's disease, *38-39*, 91, 134, 137
Pattern recognition, 30, 118-119, *133*
Pavlov, Ivan, 114
Pellagra, 82
Penfield, Wilder G., 35
Peripheral nervous system (PNS), 22-23
    See also Autonomic nervous system
Pharmacology, 134
Phobias, 95, 98
Phrenology, *134-135*
Pieron, Henri, 56
Pineal gland, 61
Pituitary gland, *17*, *23*, 24, 26, 92, 93
    Sexual behavior, 40, 42
Pleasure, 81
    Risktaking, 93, *104-105*
    See also Endorphins
Pons, *17*
Positron emission tomography (PET), 46-48, *46-47*, 87, 120
Post-traumatic stress disorder, 95
Posture, 37
Premotor cortex, 37
Presynaptic terminal, *21*
Procedural knowledge, 109, 112-114
Progesterone, *41*, 42
Proprioception, 37
Psychological disorders, 79, 82, *86*
    Sexual behavior, 43
    Whitman, Charles, 76
    See also Depression; Stress
Psychometrics, 130

Psychotherapy, 87, 95, 98
Puberty, 42, 118

R

Raphe nuclei, 60, 72, 83
Rational behavior, 126
Receptors, *21*
    Photo receptors, 28-29
    Sensory, 27, 37
Reflex actions, 23, *24-25*, *92*-93
REM behavior disorder, 67, 72
REM sleep, 56-57, 62, 66
    Dreaming, 66
    Muscle control, 57, *62*, 67, 72
    See also Dreaming
Repression mechanisms, 56
Reserpine, 83
Reticular formation, 53, 60, *72*
Retinas, 28
Rimsky-Korsakov, Nikolai, 31
Risktaking, 93, *104-105*
Roffwarg, Howard, 72

S

Schizophrenia, 53, 86, 87, 91, 134, 139
Seasonal affective disorder (SAD), 86
Sensitization, 114
Sensory receptors, 27
Sensory systems, 27-28, 126
    Neural pathways, 54
    Sexual behavior, 42-43
    Synesthesia, *30*, 31
    See also Hearing; Smell; Somatic senses; Taste; Vision
Septum, 78, 80-81
Serotonin, 60, 72, 83, 86
Sex roles, *42-43*
Sexual behavior, 40-43
Sexual dimorphism, 40-43, *42-43*
Shakespeare, William:
    Quoted, 63, 79
Shift workers, 62, 65
Sight. *See* Vision
Sign language, 118, 121, 124
Sleep, 50-52, 56-67, *60*, *61-63*
    Brainwaves, 55, 57, 66
    Circadian rhythms, 60-63, 65, *74-75*
    Deprivation, 63, 72
    Disorders, 60, 63-67, *68-69*
    Napping, *74-75*
    Non-REM, 57, 60, 66, 67
    REM sleep, 56-57, 62, 66, 67-73, *72*
    Stages, 57, *60*
Sleep apnea, 66, 69
Sleep laboratories, 50, *74-75*
Sleepwalking, 66-67
Smell, 28, 31-32
    Emotions, *31*
    Sexual behavior, 32, 42
    Taste and, *28-29*, 30
Snails:
    Aplysia, 106, 113-115, *114-115*
    Hermissenda, 114
Somatic nerves, 22-23

Somatosensory cortex, *16-17*, *32*, *33*, 35
Sound, 28
Speech, 33, 36
    Broca's area, 119, *120*
Sperry, Roger, 55-56
Spinal reflexes, 23
Split-brain operations, 55-56, *122-123*
Static labyrinth, 33
Stress, *90*-95, 98
    Type A people, 26
Striatum, *98*
Subliminal awareness, *56-57*
Substantia nigra, 38, 91, *98*
Suprachiasmatic nuclei, 60, 61, 65
Sympathetic nervous system, 24, 26, *92*
Synapses, 20, 21-22, 99, 100, *101*, 102
Synaptic cleft, 21-22, *21*, *101*, *102*
Synaptic vesicles, *21*, 102
Synesthesia, *30*, 31

T

Taste, 30-31
    Smell and, *28-29*, 30
    Winetasting, *28-29*
Temperature control, 60
Temporal judgment, 126
Temporal lobe, *16*
Testosterone, 40, *41*, 42, 43
Thalamus, 27-28, 53, 80
Thompson, Dr. Charles, *110-111*
Thought, 106, 122-129, *122-123*, *128-129*
    Neurons, *126-127*
    Sleep, 57, 60
    Spatial ordering, 119, 124
    See also Intelligence
Three Mile Island nuclear accident, 62
Tobacco, 100, 103
Twins, 132-133
Type A people, 26

U-V

Unconscious, 50, 52
    Conscious control, *58-59*
    Freud, Sigmund, 56
    Stress, 95
Union Carbide chemical accident, 62
Ventral tegmental area, 91, *98*
Vestibular labyrinth, 33
Vision, 28-30
    Color, 28
    Iconic memory, 30, 112
    Language perception, 119
    Laterality, *27*, 29-30, 119, *88-89*
    Perceptual challenges, *26*
Visual cortex, 28, 30, 126

W-Y

Watson, James, 139
Weight control, 26
Wernicke, Karl, 119
Wernicke's area, 119, *120*
Whitman, Charles, 76
Winetasting, *28-29*
Yogis, *58-59*

PICTURE CREDITS

Multiple credits on a page are read left to right, top to bottom, divided by semicolons.

Cover: Illustration by Sam Montesano with a photograph by Howard Sochurek/Medichrome.

6 Francis Leroy/Masterfile; Eric Grave/Photo Researchers Inc. 7 NIH/Rainbow; Dr. Mony de Leon/Peter Arnold Inc. 8 Red Thread Studios. 9 Petit Format/Photo Researchers Inc.; Lennart Nilsson from *BEHOLD MAN*, Little, Brown & Co. 10 Andrew McKim/Masterfile; Petit Format/Photo Researchers Inc. (4); Biophoto Associates/Masterfile. 11 Lennart Nilsson from *Behold Man*, Little, Brown & Co.; Manfred Kage/Peter Arnold Inc. (2) 12 Dr. Mony de Leon (2); M. Abbey/Photo Researchers Inc. 13 Mark MacLaren; Dr. Arnold B. Scheibel (3). 14-15 CNRI/Photo Researchers Inc. 18 Manfred Kage/Peter Arnold Inc. 24-25 Jean-Pierre Boulme/AllSport/Vandystadt (3). 28-29 John Cook (2). 30-31 Dennis Stock/Magnum Photos Inc. 33 British Museum (Natural History). 34 Dan Helms/Duomo; Don Fawcett/Photo Researchers Inc. 37 Manfred Kage/Peter Arnold Inc. 38-39 Howard Sochurek (2); Dr. Dennis Dickson. 40 Lennart Nilsson from *Behold Man*, Little, Brown & Co.; David Parker/Photo Researchers Inc. (2). 44-45 Dan McCoy/Rainbow; Howard Sochurek. 46-47 Dan McCoy/Rainbow; NIH/Photo Researchers Inc. 48-49 Al Harvey (2). 50-51 John Foster/Masterfile. 52-53 David Hockney. 57 Philip C. Jackson (6), ©1973 Warner Bros. Inc. and Hoya Productions Inc. All Rights Reserved. 58-59 Jehangir Gazdar/Woodfin Camp & Assoc.; Hartley Film Foundation. 61, 62-63 Ted Spagna. (10). 66-67 Fil Hunter (3). 74-75 Thomas Ives. 76-77 Jay Maisel. 84-85 Ed Homonylo (2), images generated by Key Molecular Corp. 87 Dr. John Mazziotta/UCLA. 88-89 The Bettmann Archive (3). 92 Philip C. Jackson. 95 CNRI/Photo Researchers Inc. 96-97 Lamb & Hall courtesy Noritsu America Corporation, creative by Marc Deschenes and Yvonne Smith. 99 Ed Homonylo (2), images generated by Key Molecular Corp. 102 CNRI/Photo Researchers Inc. 104-105 Walter Hodges/First Light. 106-107 John Allison/WQED Science Effects. 109 Dr. Robert Livingston. 110-111 Keith Philpott (2). 114-115 Jonathan Levine. 116-117 Dr. Bert Freeman; Dr. Mony de Leon/Peter Arnold Inc.; Dr. Douglas Miller (2). 118-119 Douglas E. Walker/Masterfile; Benjamin Rondel/Masterfile. 127 SIU/Peter Arnold Inc. 128-129 Courtesy Rowland Emett and Chris Beetles Ltd., St. James's, London. 133 Reprinted from *A Mensa ® Puzzle Book* by Victor Serebriakoff, International Chairman of Mensa, with the kind permission of American Mensa, Ltd. 1990. 134-135 Culver Pictures; Howard Sochurek. 136-137 Alan Carruthers; The Johns Hopkins Medical Institutions. 138-139 CNRI/Photo Researchers Inc.; Biophoto Associates/Photo Researchers Inc.; Dan McCoy/Rainbow.

ILLUSTRATION CREDITS

8-13 Josée Morin. 16-17 Sam Montesano. 18-21 Luc Normandin. 22 Sam Montesano. 23 Luc Normandin. 28-29 Robert Monté. 42-43 Guy Charette. 68 Ralph McQuarrie/Byron Priess Visual Publications. 70-71 Suzanne Duranceau. 78 Sam Montesano. 80-83 Alain Longpré. 112-113 Josée Morin. 121 Hiroko Okato. 131 Suzanne Duranceau.

ACKNOWLEDGMENTS

The editors wish to thank the following:
Addiction Research Foundation of Ontario, Toronto, Ont.; Dr. David Bloom, Douglas Hospital, Verdun, Que.; Dianne C. Brown, American Psychological Association, Washington D.C.; Peter L. Carlen, Addiction Research Foundation of Ontario, Toronto, Ont.; Dr. Neil Cashman, Montreal Neurological Institute, Montreal, Que.; Vincent F. Castelucci, Institut de Recherches Cliniques de Montreal, Montreal, Que.; Dr. William T. Couldwell, Department of Neurosurgery, University of Southern California, CA; Mony J. deLeon, NYU Medical Center, New York, NY; Patricia Dobkin, Douglas Hospital, Verdun, Que.; Frank Farley, University of Wisconsin, Madison, WI; W. Einar Gall, The Neurosciences Institute, New York, NY; Jim Henry, Department of Physiology, McGill University, Montreal, Que.; Barbara E. Jones, Department of Neurology and Neurosurgery, McGill University, Montreal, Que.; Dr. Harold Kalant, Addiction Research Foundation of Ontario, Toronto, Ont.; Leonard Lessin, New York, NY; Rajan Mahadevan, Department of Psychology, Kansas State University, Manhattan, KS; Dr. Joanne Martial, The Community Psychiatric Centre, Verdun, Que.; Dusica Maysinger, Department of Pharmacology and Therapeutics, McGill University, Montreal, Que.; Jack McCubbin, CTF Systems Inc., Port Coquitlam, B.C.; Nathalie McIntosh, Montreal, Que.; Dr. Wallace .Mendelson, Department of Psychiatry, New York State University, New York, NY; Shari Miller, Division of Medical Genetics, Royal Victoria Hospital, Montreal, Que.; Brenda Milner, Montreal Neurological Institute, Montreal, Que.; Margaret L. Moline, Department of Psychiatry, Cornell Medical Centre, White Plains, NY; Stephen H. Pasternak, Montreal Neurological Insitute, Montreal, Que.; Rémi Quirion, Douglas Hospital, Verdun, Que.; Yves Robitaille, Montreal Neurological Institute, Montreal, Que.; Dr. Norman E. Rosenthal, National Institute of Medical Health, Bethesda, MD; J. Stewart, Department of Psychology, Concordia University, Montreal, Que.; Charles P. Thompson, Department of Psychology, Kansas State University, Manhattan, KS; Lisa M. Trombetta, American Mensa Ltd., Brooklyn, NY; Dr. Daniel R. Wagner, Institute of Chronobiology, New York Hospital, White Plains, NY; Dr. Jeffrey C. Weinreb, Division of Magnetic Resonance Imaging, NYU Medical Centre, New York, NY; Sharon A. Welner, Department of Psychiatry, McGill University, Montreal, Que.; Roy A. Wise, Department of Psychology, Concordia University, Montreal, Que.; Alfred P. Wolf, Department of Chemistry, Cyclotron-PET Program, Upton, NY; Steven Zendell, Institute of Chronobiology, New York Hospital, White Plains, NY.

The following persons also assisted in the preparation of this book:
Nyla Ahmad, Elizabeth Cameron, Megan Durnford, Shirley Grynspan, Stanley D. Harrison, Jenny Meltzer, Fran Slingerland, Shirley Sylvain, Dianne Thomas.

This book was designed on Apple Macintosh® computers, using QuarkXPress®
in conjunction with CopyFlow® and a Linotronic® 300R for page layout and
composition; Stratavision®, Adobe Illustrator 88® and Adobe Photoshop® were
used as illustration programs.

Time-Life Books Inc. offers a wide range of fine recordings,
including a *Rock 'n' Roll Era* series.
For subscription information, call 1-800-621-TIME, or write
TIME-LIFE MUSIC, P.O. Box C-32068, Richmond, Virginia 23261-2068.